MODIFICATION OF THE MOTHER-CHILD INTERCHANGE IN LANGUAGE, SPEECH, AND HEARING

MODIFICATION OF THE MOTHER-CHILD INTERCHANGE IN LANGUAGE, SPEECH, AND HEARING

by

Gillian Clezy

School of Communication Disorders
Lincoln Institute of Health Sciences
Carlton, Victoria
Australia

with chapters by

Ronald J. Balthazor
Department of Communicative Disorders
California State University
Northridge, California

and

Michael J. Cevette
Combined Communication Disorders Services
The University of Oklahoma Health Sciences Center
Muskogee, Oklahoma

Foreword by
Philip S. Dale

University Park Press
Baltimore

UNIVERSITY PARK PRESS
International Publishers in Science, Medicine, and Education
233 East Redwood Street
Baltimore, Maryland 21202

Copyright © 1979 by University Park Press

Typeset by American Graphic Arts Corporation.
Manufactured in the United States of America by
The Maple Press Company.

Cover design by Jane E. Lee.

Library of Congress Cataloging in Publication Data

Clezy, Gillian.
  Modification of the mother-child interchange in language,
speech, and hearing.

  1. Speech therapy for children.   2. Children—language
3. Mother and child.   4. Communicative disorders
in children.   I. Balthazor, Ronald J., joint author.
II. Cevette, Michael J., joint author.
III. Title.
RJ496.S7C57   616.8'55   78-23352
ISBN 0-8391-1319-6

Contents

Foreword

What relevance does research on normal language development have for the understanding and treatment of abnormal development? Historically the study of normal and disabled language development has been conducted in separate disciplines with little communication between them. In the past 15 years or so, the chasm has been at least partially bridged, although the traffic thus far has been largely one way: ideas from the study of normal language development have been applied to the disabled. Considering the great theoretical importance of disorders for understanding basic processes of development, the time is overdue for some traffic to move in the other direction.

There are numerous aspects of knowledge about normal development that are potentially applicable to clinical practice. Many researchers and clinicians have been intrigued by the relatively uniform sequences of development observed in many areas of language development. These sequences provide a fruitful framework for the design of assessment instruments. It has even been argued that they provide the best guide for sequencing the content of therapy. Others have been interested in research on the role of such processes as imitation and expansions in normal development.

Gillian Clezy has taken a very different, and I believe extremely promising, tack in this book. We know that language develops in a social context. Research on adult-child speech has shown that this is a context with some fairly special properties in all aspects of language: phonology, syntax, semantics, and pragmatics. Difficulties in language acquisition may be caused or aggravated by the failure of mother-child interaction (the conventional, but occasionally misleading term for caregiver-child interaction) to occur appropriately. Sometimes this failure may be because of the caregiver's own situation or personality, e.g., anxiety about parenting and child development; in other cases it may be an understandable response to a handicapping condition of the child. But, in any case, it is the interchange that is the proper focus of intervention. The fundamental rationale for this approach, stated succinctly at the beginning of Chapter 4, Part 2, might be restated as: *conditions that are sufficient for language learning in normal children are likely to be necessary for language-disabled children.* Among these necessary conditions are the importance of meaning, rather than form in communication; an emphasis on positive reinforcement as motivation rather than selective reinforcement as a teaching tool; and, above all, a responsiveness on the part of adults interacting with young children. As Clezy points out, there are other strong arguments for using the caregiver as therapist: efficiency, greater knowledge of the child, and greater motivation.

Clezy's book is responsive to some other important trends in the study of child development. Probably the most important of these is a loosening of what is considered scientific methodology. The highly structured and generally artificial settings characteristic of laboratory work are extremely useful for many purposes, but there are many questions for which only the observation of relatively natural, spontaneous behavior can provide the necessary evidence. Children may produce behavior in the laboratory or clinic that does not occur in other settings; conversely, in many cases children can show us best what they can do when they are free to discuss a topic of their own choosing in their own way. This point applies to clinicians as well as to children. In the Introduction to Part 2, Clezy provides an eloquent argument for the observation and recording of therapy sessions as a data base for a science of clinical practice.

As more is learned about the social context of language acquisition, new hypotheses about language therapy can be formulated and evaluated. The reader is likely to disagree with some of the specific points in the present book; one of the book's merits is that it is forthright and the authors are unafraid to take a stand. For example, I believe the evidence is less than convincing that use of the visual modality for both communication and general cognitive development is debilitating to either. This book is above all an invitation to begin to approach the process of language therapy as inherently social and communicative. If language learning is interactive and creative, then so is the development of clinical practice. This analogy is well demonstrated in the final chapter, in which Clezy points out that interaction with students in the training process can have substantial benefits for the practicing clinician.

There are many other useful aspects of the book, including an admirably short, clear, and encouraging guide for parents (Chapter 4, Part 1), and a comprehensive yet introductory review of hearing assessment and amplification and their problems (Chapter 2, Part 2) well worth recommending to students and professionals outside the area of audiology.

Philip S. Dale, Ph.D.
Associate Professor of Psychology
University of Washington
Seattle, Washington

Preface

The seeds that generated this book were undoubtedly sown in my earliest years as a student speech therapist and have continued to grow throughout 20 years as a practicing clinician, predominantly in a general hospital environment, where I have been confronted with communication disorders of many and varied types.

One of the earliest questions I asked myself, along with many others, was *Why do some therapists manage to "cure" patients with complex disorders so quickly, while other struggle on with apparently simple substitution problems for years and with little apparent mutual pleasure for either patient, clinician, or parent?* I observed that, despite the fact that I was being programmed toward specific goals and objectives in therapy and toward highly specialized testing procedures and reinforcement schedules, frequently the clinics in which I saw such practices enforced were not the ones in which therapy advanced most readily. There seems to be a hidden factor, an x variable. It is not suggested that all of us who practice are not aware of such a variable. Perhaps we call it "empathy," but there is more to it than that.

Very early in my years of practice, I was fortunate enough to work with two young teachers of the deaf, who were apparently fighting the tide of tradition and had just about dispensed with all the theories I had ever heard of in relation to the young, partially hearing child. Daniel and Agnes Ling taught in the homes not the clinic; they taught the parent not the child, and they used the normal interaction between the normal mother and the normal child as the basis for all their practices. Let it be said that I did not appreciate these factors as such at the time. Conversely, I had learned to keep the parents out (they upset the child's behavior), and I saw the child's or parent's problem as something that had to be "fixed" through my interaction with him. It took but a short space of time to realize who was progressing more productively against unprecedented odds . . . the two teachers of the deaf, historically my "sworn enemies"!

Later I became a mother, and, like so many of us with the proverbial "little bit of knowledge," I looked for problems in my "risk-factor" child. It was not long before they presented themselves, I felt sure, as a developmental visuomotor disorder. There followed 10 years of evaluation as to how our anxiety manifested itself in our behavior as a family toward this apparently minor problem. The search for help began. Each time the result was the same, at least until recently. The child was assessed apart from us. The problem was always labeled visuomotor; the guidance received as to how to help in our day-to-day regime was always "nil." The weeks after the diagnostic visits, whether to the local GP, psychologist, or pediatrician, were always followed by a change in behavior on my part toward the child. I became an aggressive disciplinarian and reduced play and love time. I talked less but worried endlessly, while he became quiet and withdrawn. Friends and relations continually asked, "Well, you're worried; what are you going to do?" This in its turn, prompted the next consultative visit, which usually occurred just as I had begun to relax and enjoy myself once more with my child, and so the cycle was repeated. The visuomotor problem has nearly outgrown itself, but what of the toll upon interactive behavior? Those scars will remain forever.

I do not intend to suggest in this text that the ideas propounded are original or new. Recently I had the opportunity for a protracted spell of post-graduate study. The relief from clinical pressures allowed for time to follow interests that had been somewhat repressed, and with this came the opportunity to study researched theories from varying disciplines, some of which had formerly only been pet "hunches" to me, tried in my own practice. In a sense, many of the texts that will be mentioned herein come from fields allied to speech and language pathology. Linguistic texts, behavioral texts, audiological studies, and theories on the managment of voice, learning, stuttering, language, articulation, and behavioral programs all contribute to the vast array of published research. Few texts, however, have been written with a multidisciplinary basis for and approach to the practice of speech and language pathology. This book is a small attempt at such an approach.

Gillian Clezy

Acknowledgments

My profound thanks to my co-authors for encouraging me to put pen to paper and for sharing the task with me throughout.

To Professor Dale of the University of Washington, my thanks are due, not only for the foreword he has so kindly written, but for his interested perusal and criticism of the initial draft. His ideas, encouragement, and guidance have been of inestimable value.

My gratitude is extended to Professors Daniel and Agnes Ling of McGill University, who not only helped shape my clinical ideas as a newly qualified therapist, but also read the initial draft and gave me the encouragement, so needed, to continue.

My closest friend, Jane Lee, is responsible for the figures, diagrams, and cover design, and I thank her sincerely for her enthusiasm, skill, and interest.

To many of the staff of Lincoln Institute and Dandenong Hospital I owe my thanks for their cooperation, but particularly to Dr. Cindy Gallois for her help with the statistical analysis.

A special award should be given to Miss Marian Mooney for her courageous interpretation of the original scrawl and her typing of the initial draft and final manuscript. To Mrs. Gwenda Legg thanks, also, for her share in the typing.

Acknowledgments must go to the *British Journal of Disorders of Communication* for allowing me to reproduce some of the original work herein.

Above all, my thanks go to my sons, Mark and Bruce, for bearing with me and for providing the source of drive and inspiration with which I wrote this book.

To all the children and their mothers
who sought my help and thereby taught me;
and to all students
for whom this was originally prepared.
Above all, thank you, Mark and Bruce,
for trying to teach me to be a mother.

PART 1
THEORETICAL BASIS AND CLINICAL PRACTICUM FOR MODIFYING THE MOTHER-CHILD INTERCHANGE

Introduction

An Argument for the Reappraisal of Traditional Therapeutic Procedures

Few speech pathologists or clinicians from any discipline will argue with the fact that there is a constant need for change and adaptation in the practice of their profession. In the past twenty years since Chomsky's (1957) theories were first published, linguists have provided a wealth of research into childhood language development. Allied fields, such as audiology, neurology, psychology, and psychiatry, have also contributed to the corpus of knowledge from which the alert clinician should draw if therapy of an optimum standard is to be administered. However, in many instances adaptation is not readily accepted and traditional methods are rigidly adhered to, to the detriment of all concerned. The newly acquired knowledge, therefore, stagnates while conservative and rigid methods gain new strength. This theory has been soundly argued by Zubrick (1976), in regard to student training and research presentation, and by Ling (1976), in regard to the management of the partially hearing child. Hundreds of texts argue the same point, yet in clinics throughout the English-speaking world traditional methods are still adhered to.

What are these traditional methods? What is it that this volume seeks to adapt, negate, modify, or expand?

Traditional methods classify the speech- or language-impaired child according to medical etiology, which presupposes that the treatment will change according to the etiology. As Bangs (1968) has pointed out, this is not necessarily so. Once a global diagnosis is made and the child is accordingly labeled, a specific assessment or diagnostic procedure is initiated. The results of this procedure determine the ensuing treatment, which is carefully planned and documented with regular periods of reassessment until the ultimate prognostic goal is achieved. During the course of therapy, the child is brought to the clinic at varying intervals, which unfortunately are sometimes determined by the workload of the clinician rather than the needs of the child. Frequently, it is the parent or substitute caregiver who brings the child, and after one or two initial interviews and possibly an observation session, the parent is asked to remain outside the clinic while treatment is in progress. At the end of the session, the parent is invited in for discussion with the therapist, and a home practice program is given for use in the intervening period before the next therapeutic session.

The assumption of this therapy format seems to be that a "cure" of the disorder can only be brought about by modification of the child's behavior. He is therefore treated at a symptomatic level, and the only underlying cause that is acknowledged is the "medical" etiology. Even if the cause of the language disorder is thought to be behavioral or emotional, the child is probably treated symptomatically and referred for further assessment by personnel in allied fields, where a similar child-dominated approach may be adopted. The obvious exception to this practice is the child guidance counseling techniques in which the whole family is involved, but it is not yet apparent that such techniques have found a place in the speech pathologist's clinical battery.

Therefore, if we accept that this "traditional," child-centered approach is adequate, we also assume that the linguistic and mutually reinforcing interactions between the child and his environment, and between the mother and the child are of little importance to therapy techniques. Recent research, however, has clearly identified many areas that are critical to child development and language. Piaget's research into cognition as described by Ginnsberg and Opper (1969), the many studies discussed so clearly by Dale (1976) on the linguistic role of the mother in childhood language development, and the veritable bombardment of data concerning the detrimental effects of stress and anxiety on our lives are all vital factors apparently ignored by the traditional model.

Many therapists will argue that of course they have a full awareness of these factors, and even with the most traditional approaches speech therapy does work and children do improve. We do provide counseling sessions, problems other than the speech itself are discussed, and modification frequently results. Any clinician will be familiar with endless counseling sessions on problems ranging from nail biting and bed wetting to brother bashing and sheer defiance, but this is not enough. If current practice is to develop at the rate that research findings indicate, then clinicians must be ready to expand and develop their expertise to incorporate such knowledge. The following text is, therefore, one clinician's suggestion about how we may begin to adapt some current findings and incorporate them into our clinical regime.

The main difference between the approach expounded here and the traditional approach is that the mother becomes the "agent" of therapy. Assessment, diagnosis, and treatment plans include the search for and remediation of the clinical mother, of the clinical child, and of the clinical interactions between the mother and child. (By "clinical mother" and "clinical interactions," we mean mothers whose attitudes and behaviors need modifying and the resultant interactions which also need adjustment.) The very fact that the mother is included becomes beneficial not only for the total remediation of an interactive skill but also for two interesting side effects. First, the mother fulfills the role of clinical aide and has far more motivation to succeed in her task than those employed officially in this capacity, despite the lack of financial remuneration! Second, the mother acquires a knowledge of processes important to the development of children as a whole, and this she may generalize to other children within the family or even to the community at large. No longer does it seem realistic in the eyes of this clinician to guard the discipline's knowledge jealously against possible misuse or maladaptation, but rather it would be more realistic to attempt to educate the populace in general toward the goals that research has indicated are necessary before optimum language development can take place. Furthermore, the need at present for a healthy language environment far outstrips the supply that clinical establishments are able to offer.

As a final underlying rationale for this text, it must be remembered that the current student of speech pathology is trained to read and to evaluate research literature, but frequently does not see the literature utilized extensively in the clinical part of his training. Conversely, the practicing clinician has little time to follow the mass of research except in her own speciality, and a dichotomy of thought and terminology builds up. Despite the fact that the clinician has years of valuable experience and expertise upon which to draw, she is unable to bridge the gap with which she feels the new terminology threatens her. Only when this polarization is avoided will current research and practice produce the highest level of clinical management for the language-disordered child, parent, or situation.

SUMMARY

Research in speech pathology and allied fields has provided us with a wealth of knowledge in the last two decades. Traditional methods of therapy do not allow for the inclusion of the mother in the clinical regime, despite the fact that the mother and interactive situations frequently need remediation along with the child. Cognitive skills, linguistic interchange, anxiety levels, and reinforcement schedules are all seen as areas for possible modification along with the traditional approach directed toward speech and language skills. The mother or substitute caregiver needs to become an integral part of the program—an agent of the therapy.

REFERENCES

Bangs, T. E. 1968. Language and Learning Disorders of the Pre-Academic Child. Appleton-Century-Crofts, New York.
Chomsky, N. 1957. Syntactic Structures. Mouton & Co., The Hague.
Dale, P. S. 1976. Language Development: Structure and Function. 2nd Ed. Holt, Rinehart & Winston, New York.
Ginnsberg, H., and S. Opper. 1969. Piaget's Theory of Intellectual Development. Prentice-Hall, Englewood Cliffs, New Jersey.
Ling, D. 1976. Speech and the Hearing-Impaired Child: Theory and Practice. Alexander Graham Bell Association for the Deaf, Washington, D.C.
Zubrick, A. 1976. Recurrent Education in Speech Pathology. Aust. J. Hum. Comm. Dis. 4(2):164–167.

Chapter 1
The Model

THE GRAPHIC MODEL

In her initial work on the mother-child interchange, Clezy (1978) presented a graphic model around which she built her discussion. For ease of presentation this model is again utilized here (see Figure 1.1).

In the model the mother and child are diagrammatically depicted within their environment and are linked by the reinforcement channel. As explained in the introduction, the suggestion is that traditional diagnosis and therapy are aimed at only one part of the model, the child. No account is taken of the remaining areas of the model, which include:

1. The environment—its effect upon the child's cognitive development
2. The mother—her anxiety levels and language competence, performance, and interaction
3. The reinforcement channel—the mutual reinforcement schedules and linguistic interchanges of mother and child

If we accept that all areas of the model are in need of attention, both in diagnosis and in management, no attempt is necessarily being made to reject standard clinical procedures. They are, in fact, an integral part of the outline suggested. As Lee (1974) has said, "We are not minimizing the individuality of clinical types, but emphasizing the commonality of their language learning problems." This model for therapy suggests that there is a further commonality among language-impaired children, which is found in the clinical mother and in the clinical interactions here depicted.

Summary: The main areas for discussion are:

1. The child
2. The environment
3. The mother
4. The reinforcement schedules and anxiety levels

THE CHILD

For the purposes of this text, the model child is one that has Chomsky's (1957) innate capacity for language, and displays the

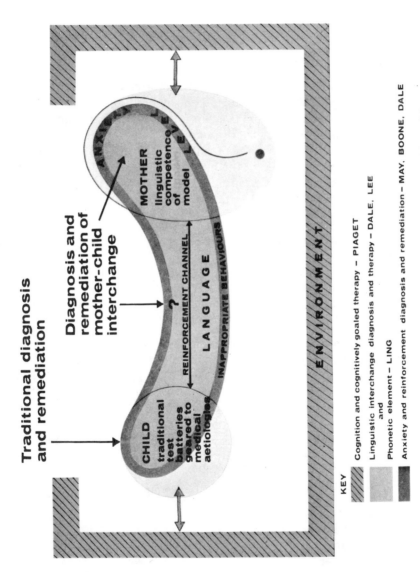

Traditional diagnosis and remediation

Diagnosis and remediation of mother-child interchange

CHILD
traditional test batteries geared to medical aetiologies

ANXIETY LEVEL

MOTHER
linguistic competence of model

?
REINFORCEMENT CHANNEL

LANGUAGE

INAPPROPRIATE BEHAVIOURS

ENVIRONMENT

KEY

Cognition and cognitively goaled therapy – PIAGET

Linguistic interchange diagnosis and therapy – DALE, LEE
and
Phonetic element – LING

Anxiety and reinforcement diagnosis and remediation – MAY, BOONE, DALE

Figure 1.1. Modification of the mother-child interchange—a graphic model.

characteristics of Piaget's "little scientist" (Ginnsberg and Opper 1969), both cognitively and linguistically; that is, he will learn primarily through his own experiences and errors, while such factors as imitation and behavior modification through reinforcement take on a secondary, but important, role.

The validity of this model is not considered here. The child is accepted as such even if preliminary investigations indicate that his innate capacity may be impaired or his self-experimenting limited through some disorder of self or of the other areas that the current model presents.

It must be stressed that the language deviant child is usually the presenting element of a language deviant situation. He is taken to the medical practitioner because he cannot talk. However, a glance through the pages ahead will show that one of the shortest sections of the text is devoted to the child alone. The assumption is that following the presentation to the referring officer, careful medical diagnosis will be carried out in the traditional manner, and either global etiologies, such as mental retardation or cerebral palsy, or specific disorders, such as dysphasia or dyspraxia, will be diagnosed by the conventional multidisciplinary team. The speech clinician will carry out her part of the diagnosis by initiating those tests of articulation and language that she feels are indicated. Having reached some form of specific diagnosis, the clinician should begin to investigate the child within the framework established by the model.

How has this child with his specific problem interacted with his environment, and how has he reinforced the persons who are his prime stimuli? Accepting that the child has this or that dysfunction, what input is he receiving? Is his inadequacy merely caused by his disorder or has the whole chain of circumstances that produces optimum language development broken down? These are the questions that must be answered, and these are the questions to which this book attends, by describing a very basic form of clinical regime that could be adapted or extended in many ways to meet individual needs.

This clinical regime is managed through the implementation of an interactive semantic and syntactic program that is similar to those used by Lee (1974) and many others. The mother becomes the agent of therapy and learns to use the skills of interaction outlined by Dale (1976). If the phonetic/phonologic (i.e., articulation) component of the language is at fault, the program outlined later and adapted from Ling (1976), using the mother as a teacher, should also be used. Both "programs" are set out as simply as possible and both allow for the mother's understanding of the steps involved and for her assessment of her own and her child's progress. The mother can achieve her own goals with the clinician's guidance, and through the use of the program she can reach an unprecedented understanding of childhood language development.

Summary: The child is accepted as having Chomsky's (1957) innate capacity for language and as having the qualities of Piaget's "little scientist" (Ginnsberg and Opper, 1969), as he develops both cognitively and linguistically. If he is a "nontalker," the initial stage in assessment, which is carried out by the traditional multidisciplinary team, should pinpoint any global or specific disorders. Further investigation before remediation should follow diagnostic assessment of the child within the parameters presented by our model.

Remediation of the deviant language is implemented by the use of semantic/syntactic and phonetic/phonologic programs with the mother as the agent of therapy.

THE MOTHER

The role of the mother is not as easily defined as the role of the child, but current research has indicated areas of prime importance, as depicted graphically in Figure 1.1.

During the early years, the mother—and by the term mother we allow for any person or persons fulfilling this role—is the provider of the environment which stimulates cognitive development. She is the arch controller of materials and stimuli, and is also the person with whom the child interacts linguistically, even from the very early months when he reacts at a receptive level. His early cognition provides him with the deep structure of his language, and the mother must interact with him as he experiments with, and develops from, the most basic elements of his grammar. We must discover if she is competent to do this and if her performance is adequate; for the mother is his linguistic model on a semantic, syntactic, and phonetic/phonologic level. If, after careful analysis, the mother's language is proved to be wanting, use of the syntactic program already mentioned will allow her to develop her grammar according to transformational principles. This can be geared to coincide with the child's developmental progress.

Last, the mother and child must interact emotionally, and we must discover if the mother's emotional status allows for appropriate and beneficial interaction with her child. The most critical factor here is neurotic maternal anxiety, as described by May (1967), which, he claims, prevents her from responding to the child's stimuli in an appropriate manner.

Each of the three roles of the mother are discussed in terms of clinical practicum at a later juncture.

Summary: The mother's role is to be the provider of the environment and of cognitive stimuli, to be the linguistic model, and to be the emotional interactor within the framework of the model.

THE ENVIRONMENT

It is not the task of this text to decide what the growing infant's environment should provide, or what is the "norm" for language development. It is, however, important that every clinician be aware that cognition is a part of the developing language, and that, therefore, before certain semantic levels of language can be reached the environment must have provided the stimuli for that language. Language can only develop as it is experienced and experimented with, as Dale (1976) has pointed out, and therefore it is unrealistic for the clinician to suppose that she can provide, within the confines of her clinic, all that is basic to the child's early cognitive and linguistic needs. To reinforce this fact, an example is given that demonstrates possible imbalance between the stimuli provided by the environment and early attempts at language teaching. Learning of some type still takes place, but it is far harder for the child to accomplish. Take the example of the 18-month-old child left in a playpen all day in his bedroom. He is cared for and loved, well fed and healthy, but his experiences are limited. A friendly aunt, a neighbor, or a clinician shows him a picture book and comments on a picture of a woman cooking, "Oh look, the mother is cooking!" During his short life, however, he has been kept away from his mother as she cooks, so that she may concentrate or so that he does not burn himself. How, then, can he experiment, and generalize from his own cognition to the visual stimuli and linguistic input with which he is now presented? He sees a picture of a woman cooking, but he has not interacted with that experience, and without doing so it is doubtful if he can conserve (Piaget, cited by Ginnsberg and Opper, 1969). Clezy (1976), in her study of 3,000 infants, observed children who were visually, kinesthetically, or aurally dominant, apparently to the detriment of the other modalities. Again we could hypothesize that this could be environmental, but further work is needed before we can ascertain whether or not such gross imbalance can be attributed to a developmental stage. It is, however, safe to assume that some mothers provide stimuli only to the modality from which they receive a reinforcing response, in which case the remaining modalities would become deprived. Does this not happen to the hearing-impaired child? To the alert clinician such examples are bordering on the ridiculous or at best on the obvious, but we must ask ourselves if we do stop to check on the environment when attempting to provide language. Furthermore do we discuss with parents the type of environment that the child has? Do we diagnose, assess, and modify the clinical or faulty environment? It would seem that the framework of the traditional model does not allow for this. Play therapy has frequently assisted the child who lacks cognitive stimuli, but also frequently the mother thinks the child just plays and is not aware of the immense significance of his experiences and his experiments. The natural, "good" mother needs no help with the environment and can frequently outstrip the clinician with ideas. The clinical mother needs help so that she does not provide a clinical environment for her child.

Summary: The clinician must be aware of what a child's environment has provided in the area of cognitive stimuli, and linguistic input should be matched to this. If the environment is found to be lacking, then modification should take place to help the child with the basic elements of his language, namely the transformationalist grammarian's deep structure and semantic component.

THE REINFORCEMENT CHANNEL

The Reinforcement channel passes between the mother and child (see Figure 1.1). Depicted within the graphic framework of Figure 1.1. are the linguistic interchange and the reinforcement schedules, both of paramount importance to the child's efforts in language.

Reinforcement Schedules

Dale (1976, citing Brown, Bellugi, Nelson, and Cazden) discusses the findings of many linguists to demonstrate that motivational reinforcement is of importance to the child's efforts, although he warns of the dangers of selective reinforcement, which will be referred to again later. As the child experiments, he needs such motivational reinforcement, but he also must reinforce his mother's efforts. If she tries to teach and encourage but gains a negative response, which is so often the case in the language-deficient child, she will soon give up. We assume herein that both the child and the mother need reinforcement at all cognitive and linguistic levels of development, and we go on to demonstrate how schedules for such reinforcement can be identified, monitored, and modified.

Language Interactions

No one can doubt that the child needs a language model—his mother—but again, as Dale (1976) points out, the role of the child is not primarily imitative but rather interactive. The normal mother expands, corrects, elicits, and qualifies her child's utterances and so adds to his linguistic experiments. She models for him as she watches his cognitive advance; she provides the symbols and "surface structures." The clinical mother may not behave as linguists have suggested the "normal" mother does, and so the linguistic interaction may become "clinical," i.e., deviant. Such interactions as there are must be observed, analyzed, assessed, and finally modified, if necessary. A perfect linguistic situation in the clinic, even if experienced daily by the child, will not match the adequate language-learning environment as a constant factor in the home.

Summary: The graphic reinforcement channels incorporate two main areas of interest:

1. The reinforcement schedules, which need to be assessed and modified to provide the maximum motivational force for both parent and child
2. The linguistic interchange, which must be assessed and compared with the norm and must again provide sufficient interactive stimuli to both mother and child

ANXIETY LEVELS

Recent research findings and many writings, among them those of Ironside (1969), May (1967), and Jersild (1968), have demonstrated that herein lies one of the major inhibitors to a mother acting or interacting appropriately with her child. Ironside (1969) goes so far as to say that the mother's anxiety affects the infant's global behavior, and prevents her from responding appropriately to any of her child's stimuli. The anxiety is generalized to the child, and a mutually reinforcing state occurs. Nijhaven (1972) found that anxiety produced aggression, authoritarianism, disciplinary behavior, and, above all, lack of communication with the child, which in turn produced states of high anxiety and behavioral traits like dependency, unsociability, tension, or lack of motivation in the child.

Presumably all parents with a nonverbal child are anxious, but the clinician must decide whether the anxiety level is "normal" or "neurotic." It could be assumed that, in the case of the latter, the parent should be referred for psychiatric management. However, if the neurotic anxiety is associated with the child's speech disorder, management by the speech clinician would seem to be the sensible approach, as she is the person who should have a deep understanding of the communication problems involved. The clinician will, of course, refer the parent on if she feels the anxiety is beyond her scope. This book suggests that it is possible to identify anxiety-based behaviors which make themselves manifest symptomatically through aggression, disciplinary comment, silence, lack of response, etc., as outlined by Nijhaven (1972). Identification of such behaviors makes their modification a moderately simple procedure, for it is this clinician's experience that the child responds quickly and so reinforces the parent toward further effort while reducing the anxiety level.

This identification and modification is carried out through the use of a Reinforcement Profile (see Figure 2.1), which is an adaptation of Boone and Prescott's (1972) category scoring technique, and which is described in detail in the next chapter. It will be noted that anxiety levels and reinforcement schedules are discussed together, as each appears to depend upon the other.

Summary: The mother of the language-disordered child is invariably anxious, and this leads to inappropriate interactive behaviors. It is suggested that such behaviors can be identified and modified through the use of a Reinforcement Profile, thus reducing the mutual anxiety levels in both mother and child.

REFERENCES

Bangs, T. E. 1968. Language and Learning Disorders of the Pre-Academic Child. Appleton-Century-Crofts, New York.
Boone, D. R., and T. E. Prescott. 1972. Contact and sequence analysis of speech and hearing therapy. ASHA 4:58–62.
Chomsky, N. 1957. Syntactic Structures. Mouton & Co., The Hague.
Clezy, G. 1976. An infant screening programme as an attempt to detect "at risk" factors for language acquisition in an Australian population. Aust. J. Hum. Comm. Dis. 4(2):146–154.
Clezy, G. 1978. Modification of the mother child interchange. BJDC 13(2): 13–16.
Dale, P. S. 1976. Language Development: Structure, and Function, 2nd Ed. Holt, Rinehart & Winston, New York.
Ginnsberg, H., and S. Opper. 1969. Piaget's Theory of Intellectual Development. Prentice-Hall, Englewood Cliffs, New Jersey.

Ironside, W. 1969. Anxiety in the Mother-Infant Interactions. World Psychiatric Symposium on Anxiety, Melbourne.

Jersild, A. T. 1968. Child Psychology, 6th Ed. Prentice-Hall, Englewood Cliffs, New Jersey.

Lee, L. 1974. Developmental Sentence Analysis. Northwestern University Press, Evanston, Illinois.

Ling, D. 1976. Speech and the Hearing Impaired Child: Theory and Practice. Alexander Graham Bell Association for the Deaf, Washington, D.C.

May, R. 1967. Psychology and the Human Dilemma. Van Nostrand Company, Princeton, New Jersey.

Nijhaven, M. K. 1972. Anxiety in School Children. Wiley Eastern, New Delhi.

Zubrick, A. 1976. Recurrent education in speech pathology. Aust. J. Comm. Dis. 4(2):164–167.

Chapter 2

Modification of Anxiety Levels Through Analysis and Adaptation of Reinforcement Schedules

The first step in the management of the language-impaired child is the implementation of traditional diagnostic procedures by the multidisciplinary team, followed by specific diagnostic test batteries administered by the speech clinician. The next step is to ascertain what the relationship is between mother and child and how it compares with the "norm." If the mother has come to a clinic with a nonverbal child, it is safe to assume that she is anxious, and it is important for the clinician to know whether this anxiety is normal, neurotic, or pathologic, as defined by May (1967). After having made some analysis of the mother's overt behaviors, the clinician has to modify them sufficiently to allow for the mother's full participation in the language rehabilitation of the child. The mother then will respond more appropriately to the child's stimuli, which in turn will reinforce his further efforts. The child's advances will alleviate the mother's anxiety, and a more healthy learning relationship will develop.

ANXIETY-BASED BEHAVIORS

Some introduction to anxiety-based behaviors has been made, but it is important to stress the critical effect it may have on both mother and child by elaborating further. Much of the current literature on anxiety describes the interactive significance of differing levels of anxiety in both mother and child. Ironside (1969) has described how anxiety in the mother has a profound effect on the infant's and the child's global behavior because of the mother's lack of appropriate responses to his stimuli. May (1967) outlines differing levels of anxiety, he accepts that a measure of anxiety is normal, but he stresses the need to modify the neurotic level. He also describes how anxiety is generalized to the child by his awareness of the disapproval of the significant persons in his world; this sense of disapproval in turn restricts his growth and awareness. Lack of advancement in the child further increases the level of maternal anxiety, and the proverbial "vicious circle" develops, which Kahan (1971) describes as "contagion." The link between anxiety and lack of communication, aggression, and authoritarian behaviors was discussed by Nijhaven (1972). Jersild (1968) has shown that childhood anger is more prevalent in anxiety-dominated situations, and that criticism and constant nagging are displayed by the anxious parent. Ironside (1969) states that negative, or even corrective, reinforcement fails to produce learning and is even stifling to a particular required behavior.

It is soon apparent that a summary of these views could be generalized to the parent who is anxious about her nonverbal child. Let us take, for example, a child who suddenly adds a new word to his vocabulary. The anxious parents are delighted and ask him to say the new word to all comers. The child, sensing an expectancy state, refuses, bringing about parental recriminations. The parental anxiety increases (they may even doubt if they have heard the new word after all), and the child's pleasure or self-reinforcement from learning is demolished or replaced by a negative attitude. An interactive schedule like this may be repeated ceaselessly in an anxiety-based relationship. Another example of such a behavior is the nonreading, learning-disordered child, who may be asked to "read" each night to his parents. His performance is so limited that it only increases the parents' anxiety, which produces further nagging and recriminations, while no positive learning takes place. Lack of motivation and tension increase in the child, and the next night's efforts become even more tortuous. If the parents could modify their anxiety to allow themselves to teach along guidelines set out for them by a remedial clinician, the whole situation could be reversed toward learning and positive mutual reinforcement.

Clezy (1976) observed in her study of infants that, even at a very early age, anxious, critical mothers apparently produced negative children with advanced "problem behavior" traits. This text suggests that it is possible to identify and to modify many of these inappropriate behaviors by using an adaptation of Boone and Prescott's (1972) category scoring technique (see Figure 2.1). The method deals exclusively with the parental reinforcement schedules elicited initially during informal play sessions.

Summary: Anxiety-based behaviors are detrimental to learning and are mutually reinforcing to both mother and child. Identification and modification must take place for a healthy language learning environment to be established.

REINFORCEMENT SCHEDULES

Before describing the Reinforcement Profile (see Figure 2.1), it is appropriate to define the level at which the vast subject of reinforcement is to be discussed. Dale (1976) has stated, as a result of other research findings, that reinforcement used selectively as a teaching device for language learning is not necessarily effective. Selectivity may, in fact, be dangerous. For example, if a child is told "No, that is wrong" when he says /ao/ for /kaet/, he may assume that he is wrong conceptually rather than phonetically. A child conceivably could be positively reinforced for saying /kaet/ correctly (i.e., "Good, you said cat properly") when, in fact, he was pointing to a dog (which the anxious parent failed to note). Such is the danger of selective reinforcement. It is therefore probably advisable, until we know more about how a child acquires his grammar and about how he balances semantic, syntactic, and phonologic elements of his language, to assume that selective reinforcement is contraindicated. Dale (1976), however, points out that positive reinforcement may be important motivationally, and if we add Ironside's theory (1969) that negative reinforcement never produces learning, it is evident that nonselective, but positive and motivational, reinforcement is of vital importance in the mother-child interactive relationship. Dale (1976) elaborates fully on how a child experiments with his language to see if the semantic, syntactic, or phonologic elements "fit" with both the linguistic and nonlinguistic situational cues he receives. If he finds that his language does "fit," it is accepted into his grammer, but if not, it is rejected. However, for all such "experiments," he needs motivational reinforcement, teaching, guidance, and stimulation. These, in turn, will produce the self-reinforcing element that results in learning.

It is obvious, not only from a review of the literature, but also from experience and observation in the clinic, that herein lies a major tool for the speech pathologist's use.

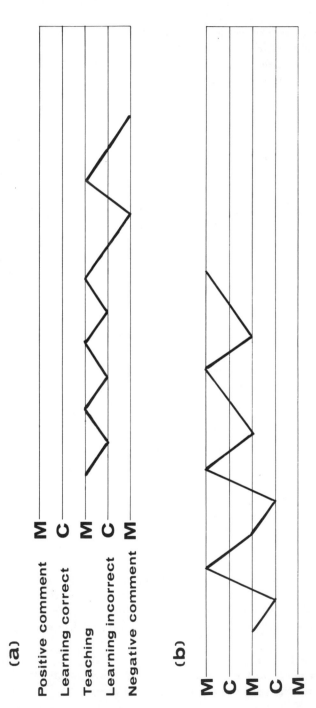

Figure 2.1. Reinforcement Profile (a) before modification and (b) after modification.

Frequently, one observes the anxious, critical mother; one might even observe the anxious, corrective speech pathologist reinforcing negatively the child's syntactic or articulation errors. This child may be struggling with the semantic or cognitive levels of his grammar, and, however hard he experiments, his efforts are being inappropriately reinforced.

If this is the environmental situation of the child, then regular visits to the speech pathologist with the anxious mother sitting outside the clinic will do little to modify the mutually damaging interchange. Involvement and understanding by the mother and progressive guidance that allows for the development of nonselective reinforcement may be the keys to a mutually more satisfying and productive approach, and hence to a lessening of anxiety. Again, the use of the Reinforcement Profile becomes the means of both identification and modification of the reinforcement schedules.

Summary: Reinforcement should be motivational rather than selective, and positive at all times, if learning is to be achieved and anxiety reduced.

REINFORCEMENT PROFILE

A study of Figure 2.1 shows that the Profile is plotted according to five different categories of interaction:

1. Teaching
2. Learning Correct
3. Learning Incorrect
4. Positive Reinforcement
5. Negative Reinforcement

These five categories are described in detail below.

Teaching

Teaching is perhaps self-explanatory, referring to verbalizations by the mother that present correct instructions, ideas, models,' or constructive questioning to the child. For example, she may give advice on some play situation; she may name an object with which the child is playing; or in a more specific teaching situation she may model a syntactic structure or particular phoneme correctly. These verbalizations are made prior to eliciting some overt response from the child.

The term "teaching" covers a multitude of specific practices, such as expansions, modifications, and modeling, and the individual clinician may find that it is more useful to break this category into smaller subcategories. This would be of particular use if a detailed individual study of the mother's linguistic practices is required. However, for identifying schedules of reinforcement, specific categories are probably not necessary, but that is for the individual clinician to decide.

Learning Correct and Learning Incorrect

Learning Correct and Learning Incorrect obviously refer to the child's responses in relation to his mother's *teaching*. Does he respond to her advice to "put the blue block on the yellow one"? Can he pick out the object she asks for or carry out the behavior she suggests? In the case of specific language interchange, we can again plot whether the response to the *Teaching* is appropriate or otherwise, and whether it is at a receptive or an expressive level. For example, the mother, working at a receptive level, names a number of objects. She then says to the child, "Where is the dog?" If he points to that animal, he has learned correctly, but if he points to the pig in response, then that response would be recorded graphically as "*Learning Incorrect.*" Having plotted the child's response, it is important to note how the mother reinforces the child's efforts. As stated before, the aim is to acquire overall motivational reinforcement.

Positive and Negative Comment

Finally, it can be seen that the Profile allows for *Positive* and *Negative comment. Positive Comment* refers to such remarks as "Good," "That's right," "Yes," "Nearly," "Good Try," and "That was nearly right." As these comments show, a mother can give positive reinforcement even when her child has made an incorrect response to her teaching. As Dale (1976) and Piaget (Ginnsberg and Opper, 1969) might say, such incorrect learning is merely an experiment to be absorbed or rejected with "cognition" or "language" according to the experimental results of the child, and should be seen conceptually by the mother as an "experiment" rather than an "error." Conversely, *Negative Comment* by the mother refers to such comments as "No," "That's wrong," "You are not listening," etc.

It may be noted that the Profile only refers to the mother's verbalizations, but it must be understood that reinforcement, whether positive or negative, can also be facial, gestural, etc., i.e., extra-verbal. Such reinforcers are not being ignored, and it is suggested that clinicians may incorporate these into the Profile should they so wish. However, it facilitates explanations to the mother if one discusses verbalizations when attempting modification, and it is this clinician's experience that, once the obvious verbal modifications are made, the extraverbal modifications follow automatically.

To elicit the behavior to be analyzed, the parent is asked to play with her child informally. This should take place after two or three visits, when both the mother and the child have relaxed and have become accustomed to the "informal" atmosphere of the clinic. Ideally, the mother should be asked to provide the materials for the play session, either from the home or from the materials available in the clinic. Close observation by the clinician should give some indication of the mother's ability to provide stimulating and imaginative material for cognitive development and matching linguistic stimulation. While the mother and child are at play, therefore, the suitability of the material (environmental stimuli) should be gauged and the chart should be plotted on the Reinforcement Profile. The clinician can then see if and when the mother teaches her child, how he learns, and how she reinforces him. She can subsequently discuss her results with the mother and initiate modification if she thinks this is necessary. A study of a number of schedules demonstrates that there is a very definite connection among teaching, positive reinforcement, and correct learning, and among incorrect learning, lack of teaching stimuli, and negative reinforcement. This, of course, substantiates Ironside's (1969) views on the uselessness of negative reinforcement.

It is here that we meet with the proverbial "which came first, the chicken or the egg?" syndrome, and it is difficult to be certain whether the correct learning stimulates the positive reinforcement or vice versa.

In the next chapter statistical information is given regarding the reliability of the Profile, and the scoring and sample analysis discussed. One of the most practical aspects of the Reinforcement Profile is that it provides the mother with a visual picture of her interactions, and she is able to "see" her advancement as she adapts and progresses according to the clinician's advice. Comparative studies are of paramount importance, and if the mother finds her own schedules difficult to modify, she may find it helpful to watch the clinician at play with her child and to plot that profile for comparative purposes. She can then try to emulate the clinician's interactive schedules. It might be suggested that the data provided by the profile are intrinsically too difficult for the mother to handle. It should be remembered, however, that these data are developed from the "normal" interactions between any mother and child, and a mother frequently has an "innate capacity" for such interaction; indeed, it is a capacity that often eludes the clinician. Even if the mother lacks teaching expertise and positive responses, her instinct and her needs seem to allow her to adapt speedily to more healthy schedules. Study of some of the profiles, particularly the profile displayed in Figure 2.1, shows the extensive modification that took place in a single therapy session. Attention should particularly be given to the entire interactive process when studying the teaching reinforcement schedules shown in Figure 2.1.

In conclusion, it seems that the Reinforcement Profile allows for a quantitative and qualitative study of the mother-child interactions and mutual reinforcement schedules, which should indicate to the therapist any areas in need of modification. By spending some time at this level of activity before language analysis and teaching, the clinician can assume that she is "normalizing" any neurotic anxieties and building a healthy foundation for further work schedules.

Summary: A Reinforcement Profile Chart, which demonstrates how the interactions between mother and child can be plotted graphically, is presented. The chart allows for discussion and modification and the recording of comparative data.

The outcome of this procedure is the development of a healthy interactive relationship between mother and child. Language therapy, with the mother as agent, can then be developed from a sound interactive basis, and the underlying anxiety can be minimized through the modification of the symptomatic behaviors.

REFERENCES

Boone, D. R., and T. E. Prescott, 1972. Content and sequence analysis of speech and hearing therapy. ASHA 4:58–62.
Clezy, G. 1976. An infant screening programme as an attempt to detect "at risk" factors for language acquisition in an Australian population. Aust. J. Hum. Comm. Dis. 4(2):146–154.
Dale, P. S. 1976. Language Development: Structure and Function, 2nd Ed. Holt, Rinehart & Winston, New York.
Ginnsberg, H., and S. Opper. 1969. Piaget's Theory of Intellectual Development. Prentice-Hall, Englewood Cliffs, New Jersey.
Ironside W. 1969. Anxiety in the Mother-Infant Interactions. World Psychiatric Symposium on Anxiety, Melbourne.
Jersild, A. T. 1968. Child Psychology, 6th Ed. Prentice-Hall, Englewood Cliffs, New Jersey.

Kahan, V. L. 1971. Mental Illness in Childhood. Tavistock, London.
May, R. 1967. Psychology and the Human Dilemma. Prentice-Hall, Engle-
    wood Cliffs, New Jersey.
Nijhaven, M. K. 1972. Anxiety in School Children. Wiley Eastern, New
    Dehli.

Chapter 3

Analysis of Mother-Child Interchange

Michael J. Cevette

The Reinforcement Profile is a five-category evaluative system. Adapted from Boone and Prescott (1972), the Profile enables the clinician to monitor the content and sequence of behavioral interchange between mother and child. The monitoring activity is easily and quickly accomplished, with the advantage that the information may be obtained from either audiotape or videotape replay, as well as from direct recording. The scoring instrument allows the clinician to quantify the mother-child interactive sequences in therapy and to record the rates of reinforcement and learning over time, so that behaviors can be analyzed, and, when necessary, modified. Clinicians must be aware of interchange rates in their therapy sessions. By monitoring mother-child interchange they become knowledgable, not only of the progress of their client, but also of what procedures lead to the most effective learning.

The following is a description of the Reinforcement Profile, and how it can be utilized to develop a more precise approach to therapy.

DESCRIPTION OF THE REINFORCEMENT PROFILE

The Reinforcement Profile is one of numerous therapy scoring instruments designed for the purpose of analyzing two-person interactions (Bales, 1950; Amidon and Flanders, 1967; Johnson, 1969; Boone and Prescott, 1972; and Schubert, Miner, and Till, 1973). Modified and truncated from the Boone-Prescott scoring system, the Reinforcement Profile utilizes five of the ten categories of the original system. The rationale for omitting the other categories from the analysis is based primarily on the behavior to be observed. The five-category system is a monitoring tool, geared specifically to obtaining information for the evaluation of the rates of reinforcement and learning. The Profile's success is founded in its simplicity. Mothers find the

Table 3.1.   Description of the reinforcement profile by category number and title

Category number	Title	Brief description
1	Positive comment	Mother-clinician positively responds to the child, either verbally or nonverbally.
2	Learning correct	Child makes a response that is correct in terms of the desired behavior.
3	Teaching ⁄	Mother-clinician attempts to elicit child behavior by direct teaching, using such techniques as modeling, statement, questioning, and expansion.
4	Learning incorrect	Child makes a response that is incorrect in terms of the desired behavior.
5	Negative comment	Mother-clinician negatively responds to the child, either verbally or nonverbally.

profile easy to understand and, also derive reinforcement and an awareness of their teaching power when they see their child's increased success rate.

The Reinforcement Profile requires the scorer to categorize a therapy event into one of five categories. Brief descriptions of the five categories are given in Table 3.1.

When rating the mother-child interchange, the scorer classifies those events in therapy that correspond to the respective categories. Three of the five categories (categories 1, 3, and 5) relate to the direct intervention of the mother/clinician. The remaining two categories (categories 2 and 4) relate to the child's performance with respect to correct or incorrect learning. Many events that are outside these five categories exist in therapy. For example, activities that comprise neutral, social, or inappropriate interchange, by either the mother/clinician or the child, may occur during the sample. The Profile does not accommodate these events, and the scorer simply omits this information from the therapy scoring procedures. Should the reader wish to evaluate these additional areas, the systems developed by Boone and Prescott (1972), or the Analysis of Behavior of Clinicians by Schubert, Miner, and Till (1973) are recommended.

MEASURES OF INTERRATER RELIABILITY

Many clinical activities rely on an observer to decide whether types of reinforcement and learning are present or are absent. No matter what the basis is for judgment, some degree of scoring error is inevitable (Fleiss, 1973). Fleiss (1975) states that, in the absence of any test that might provide a standard against which to assess the correctness of a judgment, one must rely on the degree of agreement between different judges for information about error.

In an effort to establish interrater reliability, studies of the Reinforcement Profile were conducted under three experimental conditions, two using videotape replay, where subjects scored the therapy either with or without the aid of a transcript of the test segment, and one using audiotape replay alone. Eighteen second-year students in speech pathology were equally divided among the three experimental conditions, providing six raters for each respective experimental condition. None of the students had previous experience with either the Boone-Prescott system or with the modified system.

Multiple kappa analyses (Light, 1971) for all experimental conditions showed agreement coefficients above $+0.9$. Results of the study indicated that, after a training period of 45 minutes, relatively inexperienced student clinicians can learn to independently score clinical events in therapy using the Reinforcement Profile, whether the sample be scored from videotape or audiotape replay. These data are comparable with the Boone and Prescott (1972) data that showed student clinicians learning to score their own sessions reliably using the ten-category system. After a training period of no more than two hours, live scoring results correlated 0.9 with the ratings of a panel of judges.

MEASURING SUCCESS

Precision therapy as described by Lindsley (1972), requires specification by the clinician of the tasks in the therapy session. By specifying goals and outlining procedures, the clinician can implement a program that is sensitive to the client's progress. This progress must be continuously monitored with a rating instrument that is consistent in its method of scoring and reliable in its classification. Comparisons of the information obtained from various samples of therapy over a period of time are made possible by converting that raw data into a rate of behavior per minute. Lindsley found that changes in the frequency or rate of behavior are easily read from a daily behavior chart.

As mentioned previously, both rates of reinforcement and rates of learning are derived from the information obtained from the Reinforcement Profile. A comparison of the mother's reinforcement from one therapy session to another is calculated by dividing the number of positive comments and the number of negative comments, each by the duration of the sample. In this way rates of reinforcement are established and plotted, permitting the mother to obtain a visual display of her progress.

Likewise, the child's *Learning Correct* and *Learning Incorrect* data are calculated and plotted. This provides the mother/clinician with the child's learning rate. Success rates for both reinforcement and learning are characterized by increases in *Positive Comment* and *Learning Correct* for the mother and child respectively. In the next few pages a method for obtaining and analyzing this information is discussed.

CHARTING

Lindsley's (1972) use of the Daily Behavior Chart (Figure 3.1) permits the clinician to monitor the frequency of behavior by

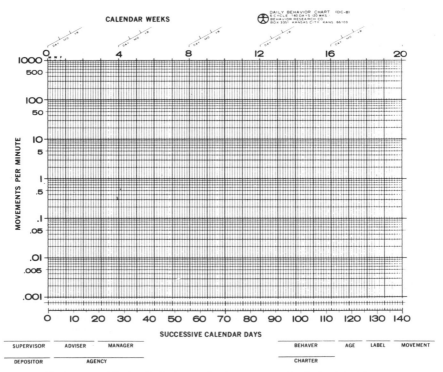

Figure 3.1.   The Daily Behavior Chart developed by Ogden Lindsley (1972).

converting raw data into a rate per minute. Conversion of the data into a visual form gives the scorer a quick impression of the changes in behavior over time. Increases in behavior, i.e., increases in *Positive Comment* and *Learning Correct*, are called *acceleration*, while decreases in behavior, i.e., decreases in *Negative Comment* and *Learning Incorrect*, are termed *deceleration*. By plotting behavior data over periods of time, the clinician and mother can quickly determine if the rate of behavior is accelerating, decelerating, or remaining stable.

The Daily Behavior Chart is a six-cycle, semi-logarithmically scaled chart and can be used for graphing one or more observable behaviors. The chart can accommodate a 16-hour (960 minutes) time sample, and a maximum of 1,000 behaviors per minute. The rate of behavior is plotted in terms of "movements per minute" along the vertical axis, which represents six exponential increments, from 0.001 at the bottom to 1,000 at the top. The horizontal axis, numbered from 0 to 20, represents weeks, and can accommodate therapy over a 20 week period. Subdivisions of successive calendar days are found within the major week divisions with the "M, W, F" representing Monday, Wednesday, and Friday, respectively. Each bold line on the vertical axis represents a Sunday. Therefore, a range of movements per minute can be plotted for up to 20 weeks on one Daily Behavior Chart. Consequently, the child's behavior rate directly influences what is presented and how it is presented. If the child's success rate decelerates, therapeutic procedures are closely examined with a possible reduction of the difficulty of the task, or increase of the strength of the cue. If the child's success accelerates dramatically, tasks of increased difficulty and/or weaker cues may be adapted. The chart provides a method for observing these changes from day to day.*

OBTAINING THE SAMPLE

Recording every event in therapy for every therapy session would be unrealistic. The analysis of the clinician's data would take more time to complete than the time required to conduct therapy. Therefore, selecting a representative sample of therapy from the total therapy

---

* Diedrich and Crouch (1972) have developed an instructional program designed to teach the speech pathologist how to use the Lindsley chart in monitoring speech and language progress.

session is appropriate. Boone and Prescott (1972) suggest recording the middle 20 minutes of therapy, and later selecting, either randomly or specifically, a five-minute sample. Boone and Goldberg (1969) have found that recording the five-minute sample will offer as much information as recording the total 20 minutes of therapy.

In another study, Schubert and Laird (1975) studied the length of time necessary to obtain a representative sample of clinician-client interaction during a therapy session. Employing as their scoring instrument the Analysis of Behavior of Clinicians System, the authors concluded that a random three-minute period from the middle 15 minutes of a 35-minute therapy session is sufficient to obtain a representative sample of clinician-client interaction during a therapy session. Schubert and Laird qualify their remarks by stating that this sample pertains only to articulation and language therapy.

For the purposes of quantifying rates of reinforcement and learning using the Reinforcement Profile, the three-minute sample has been adopted. The sample is randomly selected from the middle 20 minutes of therapy. Experience and investigation (Boone and Prescott, 1972) have demonstrated that the first five minutes and the last five minutes of a half-hour therapy session are not representative of the whole session.

A note of caution is offered, however. Boone and Stech (1970) indicated that an average of about 15% of a speech and hearing therapy session is lost with audiotape confrontation alone. The scorer will miss the nonverbal events that can only be recorded with videotape scoring. The clinician therefore should remain consistent in his method of collecting the therapy sample in order to ensure equivalent rates of behavior. Whether the clinician uses audiotape or videotape to collect data, he should replay the segment as soon as possible following the completion of the session, when the events are still fresh in his mind and more accurate recording is ensured. As suggested by Boone and Prescott (1972), playback should not be deferred more than one day.

Initially, the clinician reviews the three-minute sample with no attempt to score any event. He then scores the sample employing the five-category system. A representation of the scoring form is shown in Figure 3.2.

A check is placed on the scoring form in the category corresponding to the particular event in therapy. Following the completion of the three-minute sample, the clinician totals the number of events for each category. After totals are obtained, rates of behavior are calculated and plotted on the Daily Behavior Chart.

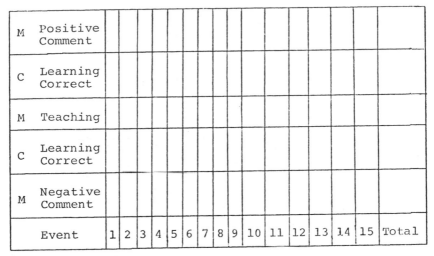

		1	2	3	4	5	6	7	8	9	10	11	12	13	14	15	Total
M	Positive Comment																
C	Learning Correct																
M	Teaching																
C	Learning Correct																
M	Negative Comment																
	Event	1	2	3	4	5	6	7	8	9	10	11	12	13	14	15	Total

Figure 3.2.   Scoring form for the Reinforcement Profile; m-mother, c-child.

Sample Transcript and Scoring

Table 3.2 is an actual segment of language therapy with a hearing-impaired child. The total time required to obtain the sample was three minutes, and following Boone and Prescott's (1972) advice, it was obtained from the middle 20 minutes of therapy. The scoresheet (Figure 3.3) and the transcript (Table 3.2) appear on the following pages.

Each event in therapy that corresponds to one of the five categories of the Reinforcement Profile is entered on the profile scoresheet by the placement of a check in the appropriate box. Following the completion of the scoring, the clinician totals the raw data for each respective category. The total for each category is divided by the time sample and a rate per minute is obtained.

Tabulation of the data obtained for the three-minute sample transcript is shown in Table 3.3. The rates per minute are plotted on the Daily Behavior Chart. Comparisons to previously obtained rates are thus made possible. The time elapsed from the selection of the sample transcript to the plotting of the obtained data is only a few minutes. The short period ensures that client behavior rates are accurately monitored.

Interactive sequences can also be plotted from the profile scoresheet. Counts of the sequence and number of learning events that are followed by reinforcement provide the clinician with information about accurate reinforcement.

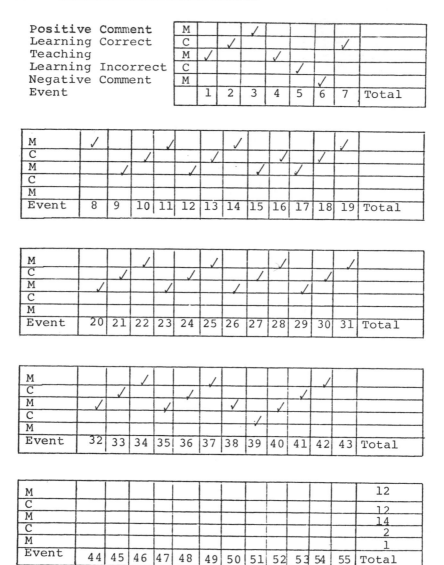

Figure 3.3.   Reinforcement Profile scoresheet showing respective categorizations of events.

Table 3.2.   Transcript of an actual three-minute therapy session with a hearing-impaired child

Speaker	Event no.	Dialogue
Clinician	1	Your car has two round black wheels. What does your car have?
Client	2	Our car has two black wheels.
Clinician	3	That's right.
Clinician	4	It does not really though, does it? How many does it have?
Client	5	Two.
Clinician	6	Not really.
Client	7	Four.
Clinician	8	That's right.
Clinician	9	But I said . . . Do you know why I said two? I said two because you drew two. What did you do?
Client	10	Drew two.
Clinician	11	Good girl.
Clinician	12	Now, how many wheels does your train have?
Client	13	Six.
Clinician	14	Great, well done.
Clinician	15	Why do you think my train got stuck? Do you know what I think? It is the train signal. What is it?
Client	16	Train signal.
Clinician	17	And when it's red, what does it mean the train has to do?
Client	18	Stop.
Clinician	19	That's right.
Clinician	20	And do you know what happened? My train got stuck, but all the other trains went rushing by. What did all the other trains do?
Client	21	All the other trains rushed by.
Clinician	22	They went rushing by. That's right. They went rushing by or they rushed on by. That's quite right. Good.
Clinician	23	Now, let's see. Your car's coming in happily and let's pretend that you met a man on a funny little red bike. You draw a funny little red bike.
Client	24	(Client draws bike.)
Clinician	25	Good girl. That's fine.
Clinician	26	What's this man riding?
Client	27	A funny red little bike.

continued

Table 3.2—*continued*

Speaker	Event no.	Dialogue
Clinician	28	A funny little red bike—uh! huh!
		Good girl. You're drawing it beautifully.
Clinician	29	He's riding the bike.
		What is he doing?
Client	30	Riding the bike.
Clinician	31	That's right. Good.
Clinician	32	And where's mummy? She is supposed to be driving the car.
		You'd better put her in.
		'Cause she's driving the car.
		What is she doing?
Client	33	Driving the car.
Clinician	34	That's right.
		Just as she drove it in this morning when you came in.
		Good girl.
		That's lovely.
Clinician	35	Mummy's wearing a brown skirt, isn't she?
		It is a pretty brown skirt.
		What is she wearing?
Client	36	A pretty brown skirt.
Clinician	37	You're a good girl and drawing it too.
		That's terrific!
Clinician	38	Well, you drew Mummy.
		What did you do?
Client	39	You draw.
		Me draw Mummy.
Clinician	40	Who drew Mummy?
Client	41	Me.
Clinician	42	You did. That's right.
		That's right. You drew Mummy. You drew her, alright, and you drew the man riding the bike and I drew the long silver train.
		So we both drew a picture and we are finished now.

Table 3.3.   Tabulation of raw data and rate per minute by category for a three-minute therapy segment

Category	Raw data	Rate per minute
1	12	4.0
2	12	4.0
3	14	4.6
4	2	0.7
5	1	0.3

SUMMARY

Precise monitoring of the mother-child interchange is an important step in the establishment and remediation of speech and language behaviors. The Reinforcement Profile, as a five-category therapy scoring instrument, enables the clinician to quantify these events of mother-child interchange.

Data obtained from the Profile, converted to a rate per minute, is plotted on a Daily Behavior Chart, which allows comparisons of behavior over time. The mother is able to view her effectiveness as a trainer, while the clinician can determine what procedures lead to most effective learning.

The use of this instrument for its designed purpose is strengthened by its reliability in rater scoring, its simplicity for mother understanding, and its effectiveness as a monitoring tool for both learning and reinforcement.

REFERENCES

Amidon, E. J., and N. A. Flanders. 1967. Interaction Analysis: Theory, Research, and Application. Addison-Wesley Publishing Co., Reading, Massachusetts.

Bales, R. F. 1950. A set of categories for the analysis of small group interaction. Am. Soc. Rev. XV:257–263.

Boone, D. R., and A. Goldberg. 1969. An Experimental Study of the Clinical Acquisition of Behavioral Principles by Videotape Self-Confrontation. Final Report, Project No. 4071, Grant No. OEG 8-071319-2814. Division of Research, Bureau of Education for the Handicapped, Office of Education. U.S. Department of Health, Education, and Welfare, Washington, D.C.

Boone, D. R., and T. E. Prescott. 1972. Content and sequence analysis of speech and hearing therapy. ASHA 14:58–62 February.

Boone, D. R., and E. L. Stech. 1970. The Development of Clinical Skills in Speech Pathology by Audiotape and Videotape Self-Confrontation. Final Report, Project No. 1381, Grant No. OEG 9-071318-2814. Division of Research, Bureau of Education for the Handicapped, Office of Education. U.S. Department of Health, Education, and Welfare, Washington, D.C.

Diedrich, W. M., and Z. B. Crouch. 1972. Programmed Instructions for the Use of Charting in Speech Pathology. University of Kansas Medical Center, Kansas City. May.

Fleiss, J. L. 1973. Statistical Methods for Rates and Proportions. Wiley Publishing Co., New York.

Fleiss, J. L. 1975. Measuring Agreement Between Two Judges on the Presence or Absence of a Trait. Biometrics 31:651–659.

Johnson, T. S. 1969. The Development of a Multi-Dimensional Scoring System for Observing the Clinical Process in Speech Pathology. Doctoral Dissertation, University of Kansas.

Light, R. J. 1971. Measures of response agreement for qualitative data: Some generalizations and alternatives Psych. Bull. 76:365–377.

Lindsley, O. 1972. From Skinner to precision teaching: The child knows best. In: J. Jordon and L. Robbins (eds.), Let's Try Doing Something Else Kind of Thing. The Council for Exceptional Children, Arlington, Virginia.

Schubert, G. W., and B. A. Laird. 1975. The length of time necessary to obtain a representative sample of clinician-client interaction. J. Nat. Stud. Sp. Hear. Assoc. 26–32 December.

Schubert, G. W., A. L. Miner, and J. A. Till. 1973. The Analysis of Behavior of Clinicians (ABC) System. University of North Dakota Press, Grand Forks, North Dakota.

Chapter 4
The Mother-Child Linguistic Interchange

There are few more clearly stated interdisciplinary overviews of the mother-child linguistic interchange than those in Dale's (1976) book, in which he reviewed the work of many others. This chapter is based almost entirely upon that work, although Lee, Koenigsknecht, and Mulhern's (1975) interactive language programs are also of vital importance. Discussing the works of Brown, Vorster, Slobin, and Brown, Dale (1976) suggests that imitation, reinforcement, and even the mother's expansions and corrections of her child's speech are not apparently the predominant methods for learning language. He suggests that the child creates and experiments, generalizes and transforms, and consequently learns and conserves primarily from his own efforts and experiments. In this he is apparently developing Piaget's theories of conservation and cognition as outlined by Ginnsberg and Opper (1969). Piaget, through his observations, associated the child's development, even to the early modification of primitive reflexes, with his concrete environment. He also described the "symbolic" years (two–four years of age) and claimed that the child will not accommodate or conserve language from narrow stimulus response situations; he needs concrete examples and interactive situations from which to symbolize. Ferguson and Slobin (1973), in their review of Bloom's work on pivot grammar and on early two-word utterances, demonstrated how these utterances are closely linked with semantic or cognitive relationships. The situation in which the child finds himself is the clue to the meaning of his utterance; it is not necessarily the word itself that carries the meaning. Only when the child has mastered semantic relationships can he learn to represent them symbolically in the form of syntax. To acquire this skill much experimenting through actions and observations is required. It is therefore imperative that the child's environment provide him with situations from which he can deduce all the semantic relationships that will later be represented by his syntactic grammar. If, therefore, we accept that conceptual relations are the basis for all developing grammar, then it is critical that the speech pathologist assess and help modify the cognitive environment where necessary. It is no use trying to teach syntax if the child has not experienced and understood the situation or relationship that that syntax reflects. One of the important skills that the parent uses in helping the child to order and process the semantic data is deixis, which is described by Newport, Gleitman, and Gleitman (1977). Deixis is the manner in which the parent indicates, either verbally or nonverbally, the cognitive cue that matches the verbal data. It is obviously an important technique.

Most important to the child, however, is the verbal language model, namely, his mother. Dale (1976) cites Vorster's findings regarding the mother's linguistic practices. The common language-teaching forms include shorter length of utterances, reduced speed, reduced number of tenses, fewer transformations, and frequent utterance of a specific linguistic structure. These and other such teaching practices have been developed by Lee, Koenigsknecht, and Mulhern (1975) into their interactive language teaching programs, which are used predominantly by the clinician. Lee et al. (1975) state that the clinical child has a reduced ability to self-discover grammatical rules, hence the structured program. Could it not be, however, that the clinical mother, because of her anxiety, has a reduced capacity to demonstrate these same grammatical rules? This inadequacy could also be generated from a lack of suitable concrete stimuli for the gauging of semantic relationships, or from a lack of normal modeling practices. A high correlation between receptive and expressive language loss and a marked effect on language by socioeconomic status and family size were found by Randall, Reynell, and Curwen (1974). These factors could be related to the above theories. For example, the lower socioeconomic group might provide fewer concrete stimuli and poorer syntactic modeling, etc. This text suggests that it is possible to analyze the mother's language practices and the child's cognitive environment and to adapt them so that they may at least approach the normal interactive situation, both cognitively and linguistically. As clinicians, we are constantly advised to adhere to the normal developmental stages of childhood, yet in one of the most normal of practices, we deviate dramatically. By tradition, we exclude the mother from the diagnostic and remediation sessions in the clinic. We build a learning environment from which the mother is set apart, and we fail to assess the quality and quantity of stimuli that she is providing.

This practice has undoubtedly developed from our lack of knowledge of the mother's role, but research has now provided us with at least a minimum of important data on the subject. For years we have known the "good" mother from the "bad," but we have accepted the "bad" mother as a necessary part of the "status quo" (except possibly in the field of family counseling and child guidance therapy). The speech clinician and other allied professionals must adapt to these new theories and treat both the clinical mother and the clinical linguistic interaction.

As a result of this philosophy, it is important to follow the identification and modification of the reinforcement schedules with similar practices aimed at establishing just what the mother's linguistic practices are. Of course, the individual clinician may decide that this can be done concurrently with the administration of the diagnostic test batteries, etc., or with the analysis of the reinforcement schedules. To elicit samples from which to analyze the mother's linguistic output it is suggested that the mother be asked to play with her child and provide the play material for the session. This writer has often been confronted with the argument that this must be unnatural for the mother and therefore must produce unreliable data. The rather negative answer to this is that it is no more "unnatural" for the mother to be coerced into a play session than it is for the child to be confronted with the traditional test battery. Obviously, the ability of the clinician to produce a relaxed atmosphere is the important variable here.

The next step is for the clinician to analyze, both quantitatively and qualitatively, the linguistic interchanges between mother and child. There would appear to be a number of ways of doing this, just as there are a number of ways of assessing a child's speech and language ranging from formal to informal testing procedures.

The use of the Profile described in Chapter 2 (see Figure 2.1), is undoubtedly helpful in that it is a *verbal* profile, at least on the part of the mother, and this writer is inclined to extend its use for linguistic analysis. For example, the Profile can provide temporal data, such as how many utterances the mother made in a given time. A breakdown of data according to linguistic principles [see Figures 4.1(a) and 4.1(b)] can provide information about semantic and syntactic content. A study of these figures will show that marked contrasts are identifiable.

Figure 4.1(a) shows a small section of interchange between a mother and her two-year-old playing with a form board. Despite the fact that the child was responding inappropriately to her stimulus questions, the mother did not attempt to teach him the correct responses. The play session, represented by the small profile, went as follows:

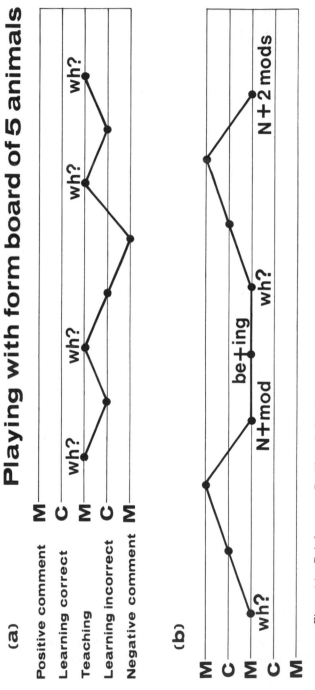

Figure 4.1. Reinforcement Profile including linguistic data (a) in need of modification (b) sample of healthy schedule.

42

The two-year-old child was presented with a form board of five animals. The mother made no attempt to demonstrate to the child how to play with it, or to tell him what the animals were; she just put the board down and said, "What's that?" (pointing to a pig). There was no response, but the child picked out a horse and a cow. The mother again said, "Where's the pig?" and the child continued to finger the cow, which brought the disparaging comment, "Don't you know?" followed by, "Which goes here?" (pointing to a vacant hole). The child, still holding the cow, inappropriately tried to fit it in, and finally the mother said very impatiently, "Why don't you look?" In a second session [Figure 4.1(b)], another parent with a slightly younger child played with the same form board, and, after demonstrating to her child how the pieces came out, the mother said, "Now, where's the dog?" (affectionately adding the child's name). Immediately the dog was found. "Oh good," said the mother, and she continued, "It is a funny dog, look how he's sitting . . . where shall we put him?" The child put him on the table and the mother said, "O.K., that's right, that's a nice big space for him." Such a procedure could, if adapted, also indicate how many times the mother was able to elicit a verbal response from her child or vice versa.

However, an adaptation of the Profile is not necessary, and traditional sampling procedures can, of course, be carried out through recording, transcribing, and subsequently analyzing the collected data. The important part is that the clinician ascertain how the mother is using length of utterance, rate of utterance, tenses, numbers, and frequency and types of transformations, and then that she compares them with normative data. All the syntactic content should be analyzed, and this can be done according to the very simplistic rules set out in the "Language Program" in the next chapter. It is also vitally important to analyze the semantic content of the sample and to ascertain if the material provided is supplying the optimum amount of concrete or extraverbal stimulation. It is difficult for the clinician not to be subjective in this particular analysis, for, as yet, research has not indicated just how much material a child can absorb and conserve. The type of material used is critical as well. Lack of interesting material, cognitively unsuitable material, boring repetition, and imitative rather than interactive situations are all threatening to the learning situation.

While the mother's speech is being analyzed, so too must be the child's. For this, of course, traditional practices may be adhered to, but let it be stressed that the interaction must also be noted. Again, it is difficult not to be subjective in suggesting the format for this part of the analysis, and standardization of interactive language tests seems but a pipe dream. However, the clinician can note, for example, who uses Wh-questions and whether or not they are answered. She can note who picks up the environmental cues and expands from them, if the conversation is significantly one-sided or lacking in balance in any way, or if deixis is sufficient and appropriate as described by Newport et al. (1977). To the experienced clinician it will soon become evident that such data are invaluable in the differential diagnosis of a particular child. For example, the mother of the partially hearing child may have reduced her utterances, the mother of the dysphasic child may be virtually silent from lack of meaningful response, and the mother of the dyslalic child will frequently repeat his incorrect articulatory patterns; all of which must be significant, even if only for subjective evaluation by the clinician.

An outline for such analysis (see Part 2, Table 5.1) is described in Part 2 of this text in the chapter on student training. It offers only a suggestion, however, and it is left to the clinician to decide what she feels should be the significant inclusions in the light of current research findings.

The stage has now been reached where linguistic diagnosis and assessment of the clinical child, the clinical mother, and the clinical interaction have been carried out. Hence, the clinician must decide at what cognitive and linguistic level she needs to introduce the language program to initiate the remediation part of the regime.

SUMMARY

If the child is to be treated within the framework of our original model, linguistic analysis of both the child's and mother's utterances should be carried out according to Dale's (1976) theories. The linguistic exchanges and formats between mother and child should also be noted and temporal factors taken into account. Extraverbal cues and material should be assessed and analyzed according to cognitive principles. Only when this has been done can a therapeutic language program be initiated.

REFERENCES

Bloom, L. 1973. Pivot grammar. In: C. Ferguson and D. Slobin (eds.), Studies of Child Language Development. Holt, Rinehart & Winston, New York.

Dale, P. S. 1976. Language Development: Structure and Function. 2nd Ed. Holt, Rinehart & Winston, New York.

Ferguson, C. A., and D. I. Slobin, eds. 1973. Studies of child language development. In: L. Bloom, Pivot Grammar. Holt, Rinehart & Winston, New York.

Ginnsberg, H., and S. Opper. 1969. Piaget's Theory of Intellectual Development. Prentice-Hall, Englewood Cliffs, New Jersey.

Lee, L. L., R. A. Koenigsknecht, and S. T. Mulhern. 1975. Interactive Language Development. Teaching: The Clinical Presentation of Grammatical Structure. Northwestern University Press, Evanston, Illinois.

Newport, G. L., H. Gleitman, and L. R. Gleitman. 1977. Mother, I'd rather do it myself. Some effects and non effects of maternal speech styles. In: C. Snow and C. Ferguson (eds.), Talking to Children. Cambridge University Press, New York.

Randall, D., J. Reynell, and M. Curwen. 1974. A Study of Language Development in a Sample of 3 Year Old Children. Br. J. Disord. Commun. 9:3–16.

Chapter 5
The Language Program

A global diagnostic regime can be adapted to suit clinical children, parents, and interactions simultaneously. If we find, after our diagnostic sessions, that all three are in need of attention, it is sensible to attack the emotionally based conflicts first, as already suggested. It is important to reiterate Ironside's (1969) theory that negative reinforcement is counterproductive to learning. The clinician intends to teach language and/or articulation, yet it is impossible for her to approach the norm of language learning as outlined by Dale (1976) unless the mother becomes the agent of therapy. It could be that the mother's language needs more attention than the child's (see Figure 4.1), and she too will need help in reducing her anxiety level and will need positive reinforcement. Schedules to accomplish this must be worked on until positive reinforcement is the rule rather than the exception. When the clinician feels that the mother and child are playing "happily," and that cognitive material is matched to the child's level of maturation, the program below can be introduced.

THE MOTHER AS AN AGENT OF THERAPY

Earlier chapters give some indication of why the mother or caregiver should become the agent of therapy. To repeat and summarize, the reasons are:

1. The "normal" child should be taught by the "normal" mother.
2. No clinical situation can provide all of the cognitive stimuli of day-to-day living, and therefore no clinical situation can provide sufficient material for language learning and conservation.
3. The mother's participation in therapy will modify her own habits, and she will generalize the new-found knowledge from clinic to home and to siblings.
4. The understanding so acquired can also be generalized to the populace.

With reference to the final point, this writer feels that there is little danger of maladaptation in the public's becoming linguistically educated. There is no danger of maladaptation if a natural procedure is the goal of the therapeutic program. Mothers and children have been teaching and learning language for years!

The building of a semantic, syntactic, and/or phonetic/ phonologic program that is within the scope of the average person's understanding is the first necessary step in planning a therapy regime for the mother. One such program is described below. It is developed from the methods Lee, Koenigsknecht, and Mulhern (1975) used but is simplified for the mother's benefit. Vorster (1974) found that mothers used fewer transformations in their utterances to their children, and he also noted a reduced rate of speech, reduced mean length of utterances, and repeated use of specific structures. This program is introduced with these skills in mind.

In the use of any program there is one grave problem: mothers do not *normally* work with a program, and we do not have proof that there is a given order to which mothers adhere as they model syntactic structures [although Lee (1974) has indicated that there are developmental hierarchies]. We know, as previously discussed, that the child works from the basic deep structures and semantically based relationships of his language, through noun phrases and verb phrases, toward more sophisticated transformations. We know that he is prompted by extra-verbal or environmental cues, which also prompt his mother to give him the linguistic model for his "researching." We know, above all, that he experiments. It is absolutely critical that he be allowed to develop in just such a manner. A program could ruin this process if simple stimulus/response learning (i.e., rote imitation) is involved. The following program, therefore, is not rigidly sequenced; it does not suggest that a child must learn one structure before advancing to the next; it does not even suggest an order in which to present the material. Most importantly, it is not imitative. The program attempts only to provide the most basic of syntactic grammars from which it is hoped the child will be able to "generate" and "transform" according to Chomsky's (1957) principles. There is no age hierarchy, no developmental hierarchy, and no aim at formal presentation. Why then do we present a program at all? It is a means by which we assess and set goals for our language teaching, and it is a means by which we can assess and teach the clinical mother. Finally, it aims at producing some specifics for therapy out of the vast mass of materials that we ambiguously call language. Possibly, our teaching would be just as effective if we gave the mother one simple instruction, i.e., "Talk to your child," but such a procedure would be insufficient for the mother with suspect modeling practices. Furthermore, when the mother is requested to simply talk, it is hard for her to evaluate her own achievements. With a program she can hear and enjoy her child experimenting with syntactic utterances that she has modeled for him. She knows "where she is going and what she is doing." The mother uses the program to elicit specific structures, but later both she and the clinician can use the material as a basis for analysis of spontaneous speech. It is this clinician's experience that most mothers can quickly analyze a spontaneous utterance that their child has made. Some common parental comments are: "He used two noun modifiers," "I heard four irregular pasts today," or "He understands six of those Wh-question things, but he only uses 'why'!"

The mother may choose how to implement the program, she may hold a target structure in her mind for occasional and random use throughout the day, or she may prefer a specific play session. There are parents who designate a particular activity as "language time," e.g., the drive to kindergarten, or the visit to the supermarket. All of these can be equally beneficial, and it is not for the clinician to stipulate what the practice should be. It is, however, important that the clinician be able to watch the interchanges in question; above all, she should see that they are interactive rather than imitative, are matched to the cognitive stimuli, and are experimentally oriented for the child. If the target structure is not elicited, negative reinforcement must still be avoided, for the child may be experimenting. The mother needs to expand the concept and to correct the child without any suggestion that he was wrong. There may be an infinite number of responses to one question that the mother hopes might elicit some structure she has modeled. Therefore, when the child does not reply with the given model, he is not necessarily wrong. If his reply is appropriate to the extraverbal cues, or indeed to the verbal stimulus, then he is right and is experimenting well, and he should receive appropriate motivational reinforcement. We cannot tell with which element of his language a child is struggling, and we must allow for this fact.

Summary: By teaching the mother the basis of a semantic and syntactic grammar, we are able to provide her with an understanding of these elements of language. She is able to modify her own utterances toward a specific structure, which she now knows is part of every child's basic grammar; she can elicit a response interactively; and she can evaluate her own and her child's achievements.

The program is not ordered and must cater to interactive rather than imitative responses. It must also allow for all the natural processes of language learning discussed in previous chapters.

THE CHILD AS A RECIPIENT OF THE PROGRAM

The role of the child in the implementation of the program should be that of the normal child in a healthy linguistic environment. No pressures should be put upon him that will prevent optimum learning. The stimuli for the discussion should be materials or activities that he has chosen, or in which he is interested. They must be cognitively stimulating and must allow for semantic development. The child should not be aware of the fact that the mother has a target structure in mind and therefore should not be required to repeat, for example, endless modified nouns without any other linguistic information. His role should be "experimental" and "scientific" and the language element should only be a part of the total experience. He must be allowed to see if what he says "fits" with the extraverbal cues and with what his mother's and his own acquired language dictates. He must be allowed to reject or accept the elicited data in his own time, and after sufficient experimenting, he should have his utterances expanded upon, his questions answered, and his statements heeded. He needs reinforcement which will motivate his further efforts.

Summary: The child's role during the language program should be that of the happy, interested participator who is allowed to experience, to experiment, and, by so doing, to learn at his own rate. He should not be aware of any specific program, but should be content in the fact that his mother is talking to him and responding well and appropriately to the stimuli that he gives to her.

A LANGUAGE PROGRAM REDUCED TO A
BASIC GRAMMAR AND ADAPTED TO INFORM PARENTS

YOUR CHILD AND HIS LANGUAGE:

1. If you have a child who is having problems with language learning, no amount of speech therapy will improve the situation nearly as well as you can as parents. Where do all children learn their language? In their home with their parents. The clinic is the place where you will learn how you can help your child.

2. Do not worry; you do not have to teach your child every single thing he will ever learn to understand and say. There are an infinite number of computations. All we have to do is to let him hear all the basic patterns, and he will do the rest by creating the sentences that he needs to suit his purpose.
3. How can you teach him all the patterns? You can teach him by chatting to him about your everyday life, and by chatting as you play or look at books. Just remember that a child will not learn words unless he understands what they mean. This is easy to achieve if words are used along with actions, things, and happenings.
4. Remember, your child does not have to say something to show that he knows it. If he listens to you, he will be learning, and he will talk when he is ready.
5. Do not worry if he does not say things properly, or as you think he should. He is like a scientist; he must experiment before he succeeds. The things you think are mistakes may just be experiments. You may prompt him, however, as you think fit; this helps the experiment.
6. Table 5.1 is an explanation of how a child learns his language. Most of this is completed between 5 and 6 years of age. If you would like to help, you can take any section, think about it, and talk to him, using that type of language. You will then be sure that he has heard that particular example, and so he should learn it. Do not try to do all sections at once.
7. Remember that children only learn if they are interested, so enjoy your "language-time," and also remember that your voice and the patterns it makes—the pauses and stresses in your speech—are just as important as the words themselves.

STAGES OF LANGUAGE:

Very young children learn single words, and they learn that words must have an order to mean something. They also learn that there are "thing" words—NOUNS—and "doing" words— VERBS. Gradually, they add to these two groups, as is shown in Table 5.1.

SENTENCES:

The child can now produce a noun phrase or a verb phrase, but there are extra things he needs to learn to produce a sentence. He must know about the word order and about subject/verb/object. Add the pronouns, negatives, and questions in Table 5.2 with the phrases that have been learned from Table 5.1.

When your child has heard and understands all such examples, he will have learned a lot of the basic rules. Just give him the chance to hear them. Ask your therapist how to use

Table 5.1.

Nouns	Parents	Verbs
Objects or things, e.g., car, dog	Show him as you *Talk* and *Play*.	Doing words—make, cook, see
Expanded into noun phrases—to do this he must know the order that he needs to use.	Show him as you cook, work, or play—talk as you do.	These are expanded into verb phrases, but he must understand in his play the difference between:
The noun can be expanded by the use of:		1. *A continuous action*—"I am doing something"
1. *Article*—a car, the car		2. *A completed action*—"I did it"
2. *Possessive*—Daddy's car	Work on one example at a	3. *The ability to do*
3. *Quantifier*—more cars	time, but in lots of ways.	*something*—"I can
4. *Adjective*—big car		play"
5. *Designator*—that car		
A number of these can be strung together, but they need an "order."		
(2) (3) (4)		*Verbs* are expanded by
Daddy's two big	Describe things with lots of	1. *Imperative*—go, walk
(4) (3)	words.	2. *All the 'be' words*—am,
blue cars		are, is, was, were
(the numbers refer to the list above)		+ *ing* "I am walking."
		3. *Regular past*—walke*d*
Dangers		(Verb + *ed*)—jumpe*d*
a. He may get the wrong order.	Stress them in your speech.	4. *Irregular past*—went, saw, did
b. He may not know the difference between "a" and "the," e.g., "a man in the street."		5. *Verb extras* (+ *verb*)
		aux: modals:
		do can
		be may
		have will
		shall
		must
		also
		Be + *have* can be main verbs
		Be—"He *is* small."
		Have—"I *have* it."
		Dangers
		The "be" words are often excluded, e.g., "Daddy here."

them, if you need to. Some extras that you might add are: negation words, e.g., nowhere, nobody, never, none, and passives.

REMEMBER—HUNDREDS AND THOUSANDS OF
WORDS CAN BE USED WITH THESE PATTERNS

In the Language Program all aspects of noun phrases and verb phrases in their simplest forms are worked on, and are gradually woven into transformational structures as learning advances. Language sampling must, of course, be carried out at regular intervals to ascertain whether or not a particular structure has been absorbed into the child's grammar.

For readers interested in acquiring the skills necessary for interactive therapy, there is no better text than Lee, Koenigsknecht, and Mulhern (1975), but to facilitate the reader, one sample of each structure contained in the above program is summarized below, with a sample interchange aimed at eliciting a response already modeled. Careful note should be taken of the child's responses in comparison with the model, and of the resultant expansion or reinforcement given by the therapist or mother. All examples are taken from actual clinical sessions.

THE ELICITING OF PARTICULAR
STRUCTURES FROM THE LANGUAGE PROGRAM

The following preparatory work should be carried out by the clinician prior to working on the given structures.

1. The language structures and general philosophy of cognition and language should be explained to the mother at her level of understanding.
2. Play materials and daily activities should be discussed with the mother.
3. Therapist and child should play together with suitable extra-verbal material.
4. First, the therapist should demonstrate to the mother how to introduce the target structure [well "padded" with other language (unless contraindicated etiologically), which is excluded below for spatial reasons].
5. The therapist should then demonstrate appropriate questions and statements that might elicit the target structure in response.

Table 5.2.

Pronouns	Negatives	Questions	Introduction of verbs + negative	Conjunctions	Infinitives
Subjective: I, you, he, she, us, it, they	Negatives can change the whole word order.	Questions change all the word order, and can be asked in lots of ways.	How does it change the verb?	But, so, if, because, or Also all "Wh" words. (see Questions)	To + verb "I want *to* go." "I know where *to* find it."
Objective: Me, you, him, her, it, us, them	The word "not" must be put in the right place:	(a) "Car?" (b) "Car, eh?" (c) "That a car?" (d) "What (Who, Where, Why, When, Whose, How, Which) is that?"	(a) "We haven't . . ." (b) "You aren't . . ." (c) "We don't . . ."	Meaning of conjunctions is difficult for the child to learn.	"He came *to* play." *Practical Hint:*
Possessive: Mine, yours, his, its, hers, ours, theirs	"Daddy is going out." "Daddy *is not* going out."	(e) "That's a car, isn't it?"	*Practical Hint:* Use this in many ways in your speech.	*Practical Hint:* Use all conjunctions appropriately with an obvious example:	Use infinitives as you look at books, etc. "The fish wants to swim."
Which pronoun to choose and *when* is very important. N.B. "The big round red ball" could be just "it."	*Practical Hint:* In play, etc., sometimes tell your child what you are *not* doing.	Change of order: "The dog is looking at us." "What is the dog looking at?"		"We'll go outside only if it's not raining, because we don't want to get wet."	
Practical Hint: Looking at pictures inspires long descriptive phrases,		*Practical Hint:* (a) Ask lots of different questions in your			

but also use sentences with "he," "she," etc. Contrast only two at a time.

play, and give the answer.

"What shall we build today?"

"We'll build a house."

"Where shall we build it?"

"Here."

"Who will live in it?"

(b) Play games about other people asking questions.

You: "The man said 'Who's that?' What did he say?"

Child: "Who's that?"

6. The therapist demonstrates appropriate reinforcers and expansions, etc.
7. The mother is asked to demonstrate a similar interactive language session to the therapist.
8. The therapist modifies reinforcement schedules and linguistic interchange appropriately.
9. The mother works on this structure at home before the next clinical visit. She does not work on one structure exclusively, but uses it on random occasions throughout the day. All her language should provide general enrichment and motivation.

Introduction of Noun + Modifier(s) or Verb + ing

Th/M = Therapist or Mother, *C* = Child

Th/M   "Look at all these toys! [*farm animals*] Can you see them all? Aren't they nice?"

Child looks, touches, explores, matches.

Th/M   "Good, Mm hm, OK." [*nonspecific reinforcer*] "Here's a brown cow. It's eating." [*target structures*]

If the target structure is Noun + Modifier:

Th/M   "What is it?" [pointing to cow]
C   "A brown cow."

If the target structure is Verb + ing:

Th/M   "What's she doing?"
C   "Eating."
Th/M   "Yes, she is, she's eating. The brown cow is eating the grass." [*expansion reinforcer*]

Note: To acquire "ordering" of all modifiers, listed noun phrases are expanded.

Introduction of Regular Past Tense

Th/M   "Let's play some doing things today."

Therapist indicates to M & C various activity corners or "stations" where each will play follow-the-leader with a particular activity, etc.

Therapist goes to corner and jumps.

> *Th/M* "Look, I'm jumping."

Therapist finishes jumping and says:

> *Th/M* "What did I do? I jumped!"

Therapist answers her own eliciting question appropriately.

> *Th/M* "What did I do?"
> *C* "Jump" [*no* 'ed']
> *Th/M* "Mm hm, I jumped, I really jumped."

Therapist agrees motivationally on semantic "jump," then repeats target structure.

> *Th/M* "You have a turn now. [Child jumps.] "Good, you jumped!" [*reinforcer and remodel of target structure*]
> *Th/M* "Now Mummy your turn!"

Mother jumps.

> *Th* "What did you do Mummy?"
> *M* "I jumped." [*repeated structure*]
> *Th* "Right, you jumped well." [Jumps again herself.] "I jumped."

Child jumps in turn.

> *Th* "You jumped, what did we all do?"
> *C* "Jumped"
> *Th/M* "Yes, we jumped, we're great; we jumped and jumped and we jumped." [*reinforcers*]

Introduction of Irregular Past Tense

> *Th/M* "Look at these lovely circus people. [*cardboard circus figures*] Have you ever been to the circus?" [*to verify if cognitive semantic material is suitable*]
> *C* "Mm hm"
> *Th/M* "I went last week. [*model, 'went'*] When did you go?" [*appropriate eliciting question*]
> *C* "I went with Mum!" [*Child gives incorrect response to 'when' but uses irregular past!]*
> *Th/M* "Lucky you" [*interest as reinforcer*]

Therapist turns to mother and repeats "When did you go?" [*to help child over semantics of 'when'*]

> *M* "Last week, we went last week." [*natural, informed parent*]

All the time the 'toys' are being fingered, touched, and arranged.

> *Th/M* "I saw some of these when I went. I saw horses. I saw elephants. [Therapist touches and moves them.] What did you see?"
> *C* "I saw these."

Child points to clowns

> *Th/M* "Did you? What did they do?"
> *C* "They maded me laugh." [*incorrect past*]
> *Th/M* "Weren't they funny? I saw them too. They made me laugh." [*expansion and correction*]

Introduction of Verb Extras (Auxiliaries and Modals)

Therapist is looking at a book.

> *Th/M* "Look at this little girl. She looks as if she wants that lolly. Do you know what I think she is saying? She's saying 'I can have it Mummy, I can have it.' Look, she's even stamping. What's she saying?" [*added material: stamping is added to avoid immediate 'rote' repetition*]
> *C* "I can have it."
> *Th/M* "That's right! That's just what she is saying. [*reinforcer*] Do you think the Mummy gives it to her?" [*expansion and continuation*]
> *C* "No, she's naughty."
> *Th/M* "Oh! Is she? Well maybe her Mummy says to her 'You must be good first.' What does the Mummy say?"

Therapist has taken lead from child's spontaneity.

> *C* "She must be good." [*not an exact repetition of 'You must be good' but absolutely correct*]
> *Th/M* "And is she good?"
> *C* "No!"

Note: Verb extras + negatives can be elicited in much the same way.

Introduction of Subjective and/or Objective Pronouns

Any variation of the Three Bears Story or adaptation thereof may be used, e.g., and the Daddy Bear said, "Whose been eating *my* porridge," etc.

> *Th/M* "Let's do some drawing today. We'll draw four people. [Th & C draw.] There, I've drawn a mother, and a father, and two children, and I'll give the father his eyes, and the mother her eyes, and the children their eyes."

Therapist watches child copying and takes cue from what the child is doing. For example, as child draws father's eyes . . . "That's his eyes. Child draws mother's eyes. What's that?"

C   "Eyes"
Th/M   "Yes—they're good, they're her eyes. [*the mother's*] Now whose are those?"
C   "His" [*the drawn child's*]
Th/M   "That's right. Now look, my poor father can't smell. He says 'Where's my nose?' because he wants to smell. You give one to *him*." [*stress*]

Child draws lots of noses.

Th/M   "Good, and to him. Yes, and to her, and to them. Well done, you gave noses to all of them. You drew their noses, didn't you? What did you draw?"
C   "Their noses"
Th/M   "Good, now they can all smell."
C   "Mm hm, but look, no hair.".
Th/M   "We'll give them their hair."

Both draw.

Th/M   "What are we giving them?"
C   "Hair" [*no pronoun, but correct*]
Th/M   "Mm hm, their hair, he's got his, she has hers, and the children have theirs."

Therapist points appropriately.

Th/M   "It's good, but it's not as pretty as yours, is it?"

[Therapist touches child's hair.]

Th/M   "Where's my hair?"
C   "There"

[Child indicates.]

Th/M   "Whose hair are you touching?"
C   "Yours"
Th/M   "That's right. That's my hair."

Note: For the difficult mine/yours, or me/you a third person is introduced as in "The Three Bears."

Introduction of Negatives

It is important that negatives be introduced progressively and be linked with the child's cognition of the negative concept. Comparison with the "positive" is obviously valuable. The discerning clinician should be able to ascertain the appropriate stage of introduction for various negative structures. Obviously, it would be inappropriate to introduce the structure "must not"—at least for expressive purposes—until the positive form has been mastered. There appears to be a hierarchy of negative structures, from the simple "no more" to the more sophisticated transformations incorporating auxilliaries and modals, or the negative interrogative reversals. The following sample includes a number of negative structures that may be introduced. Notice that some are supplied at a receptive level only. The individual clinician should feel free to expand and adapt, or simplify and reduce, according to the child's needs and responses.

> *Th/M* "Let's dress all the dolls today. [*cardboard dolls with separate clothes which can be fitted onto them*] Which one would you like? Take a look at all of them. I don't want this one. Look, he looks cross. But he isn't."

Therapist picks up another.

> *Th/M* "I like this one. I'll have this one."

Therapist hands the child a doll, inappropriate to the child, e.g., a baby girl doll for a 'tough guy.'

> *Th/M* "Do you want this one or not?"
> *C* "No—yuk. I want this, no, this one. He's a boy!"
> *Th/M* "Does he have any clothes?"
> *C* "Nope"
> *Th/M* "No, he doesn't have clothes. Is he warm enough?"
> *C* "No"
> *Th/M* "No he is not warm at all is he? He is cold. What is he?"
> *C* "Cold. I put this on."

Child excluded 'I'll put,' so therapist modifies.

> *Th/M* "That's nice of you, you'll put it on and you'll make him warm, but I don't think he'd wear a coat before a shirt and pants. It would be funny. You don't, do you? You don't put your coat on when you get up. It is not the first thing you put on is it?" [*all the time at a slow rate while exploring the 'toys'*]
> *C* "No, course not"
> *Th/M* "Of course you don't, you put on your underclothes first. Has he got his on?"

[Both look.]

> *Th/M* "No, no underclothes. Let's find them."

Both therapist and child put on appropriate clothes.

Th/M   "Now, will he be cold?"
C   "No he's warm, isn't he?"

Therapist thinks 'Hurray!'

Introduction of Questions

Note: The therapist should remember that there are a number of different types of questions, e.g., inflective questions, Wh-questions, interrogative reversals, and tag questions. For our purpose we can demonstrate the modeling and eliciting of the Wh format, but all formats can be elicited by using a third person, or spokesman, in the exchange, as in the sample below.

Wh-Questions

These questions are listed in the Program. It is wise to introduce only one or two at a time, to allow for conceptual discrimination.

Th/M   "We'll play with the doll's furniture and with this family today."

Therapist selects kitchen furniture, dining table, and table setting.

Th/M   "Look, we have a mother, father, and children, a table and four chairs. They are all going to have their lunch, but father isn't home yet. We'll keep him over here at work."

[He is placed separately.]

Th/M   "The mother is busy cooking here, and she asks the children to get the table ready. Do you help your Mummy lay the table?" [*ascertaining that the child is cognitively "in tune"*]
C   "Yes"
Th/M   "Good, well look, this little girl is putting the chairs round, but there's one missing and she says to her Mummy 'Where's the chair?'"

[Therapist is searching for it with hands].

Th/M   "What does she say?"
C   "Where's the chair—Look here 'tis."
Th/M   "Oh, well done! Now they can all sit down, but look, they don't have anything to eat. This boy says to his mother, 'What's for dinner?' He is hungry, so what does he ask her?"
C   "What's for dinner?"

Th/M   "That's right, and what do you think is for dinner?"
C   "Fish'n chips"
Th/M   "That's a good idea! Well, the mother is just about to serve it but she says, 'Where's Daddy? He should be home. Where's Daddy?' What did she ask?"
C   "She said, 'Where's Daddy,' but look he's coming."

Child grabs 'Daddy' and makes him "come home."

Th/M   "Good, he's just in time for lunch, isn't he?"

Therapist throws in a tag question for good measure.

Introduction of Conjunctions

Note: By this time the child is usually fairly competent linguistically, and it can be seen that the interchanges could be far more lengthy, particularly if "Wh" words are used in conjunction form.

Th/M   "Today we'll play this game of lotto."

Therapist produces a game with plenty of visual information, and the child has to match scenes visually, by selecting small cards that are matched to a master.

Th/M   "There, that's your card, this is mine. We'll pick these up in turn. I'll start. What have I?"

[Therapist looks at card.]

Th/M   "Oh look, he must be a clown because he's wearing that hat. How did I know he's a clown?"
C   "Cos of the hat"
Th/M   "Right, because of the hat. [*reinforcers, remodels, and places card*] Your turn, good, that's right. Good gracious another clown, and what's he got? They could be apples, or balls, or oranges? What could they be?"
C   "Oranges"

Child is quite decided, therefore did not use conjunction 'or'.

Th/M   "Oh, so you think they're oranges, well you're probably right, [*considers*] but I think they could also be apples, or they could be balls. What do I think they could be?"
C   "Apples or balls, but [*note spontaneous conjunction*] they're not. Look they're orange oranges." [*stupid therapist!*]
Th/M   "I'm sure you're right, my turn . . ."

These samples are but a few of the very many ways in which the exchanges can take place. It is not suggested that they portray all the material necessary to the child's basic grammar, nor have all the structures in the program been demonstrated. The alert clinician who is familiar with linguistic data will soon find many ways to generalize from this very basic hypothetical format. Again, the ordering is not necessarily critical, but obviously, phrases will come before sentences and plain verbs before verb extras, etc. There should be no rigidity in learning and nowhere is it suggested that one structure must be acquired and integrated into the child's grammar before another is introduced. Individual decisions about each child, and each mother, should be made in relation to the diagnostic information and observed data.

The type of play material and experiences used should be noted. During the earlier linguistic period, the materials are concrete and three dimensional, or, as with the basic verb phrase, the child acts out and experiences the language that he is hearing. Later, however, as the child advances, the material becomes two dimensional or symbolic. It cannot be emphasized too strongly that extraverbal and verbal cues must be linked and matched to suit the child's conceptual capabilities.

The structures outlined above demonstrate how one may elicit language expressively, but it is just as easy to use the program at a receptive level, at an earlier stage, or at interim stages of the child's development. There can be no marked dichotomy between reception and expression in the true interactive state. Close study of the samples will show that some of the language used could be assessed as language far in advance of the child's expressive capabilities. Herein lies the receptive element. In addition, if there are severe problems in implementing the program it may be used at a more basic level of reception. Obviously, in this case, the response to be monitored is the cognitive response or nonverbal response of the child. The latter is of great value—particularly as far as the mother's morale is concerned—in the treatment of autistic, grossly mentally retarded, dysphasic, or severely hearing-impaired children.

SUMMARY

A program incorporating a basic grammar from which the child can generalize and create, and which the mother should be able to understand is presented. The mother must first watch the therapist and then demonstrate to the therapist how she intends to play with the child and to elicit the proposed structures. The therapist should monitor and modify the responses according to all the principles already discussed. The verbal material must be presented with suitable extraverbal material, and the child's spontaneity and creativeness should be catered to, both cognitively and linguistically. For this reason, there should be no rigidity in presentation. The skills required by the clinician and mother are outlined by Dale (1976). Some of the structures contained in the program are demonstrated, but it should be understood by each clinician that there is no "set" way. The program can be adapted in many ways to suit individual needs.

REFERENCES

Chomsky, N. 1957. Syntactic Structures. Mouton, The Hague.

Dale, P. S. 1976. Language Development: Structure and Function, 2nd Ed. Holt, Rinehart & Winston, New York.

Ironside, W. 1969. Anxiety in the Mother-Child Interaction. World Psychiatric Symposium on Anxiety, Melbourne.

Lee, L. 1974. Developmental Sentence Analysis. Northwestern University Press, Evanston, Illinois.

Lee, L., R. A. Koenigsknecht, and S. T. Mulhern. 1975. Interactive Language Development. Teaching: The Clinical Presentation of Grammatical Structure. Northwestern University Press, Evanston, Illinois.

Vorster, J. 1974. Mother's Speech to Children. Some Methodological Considerations. Institute Voor Algemene Taalwetenschap, Universiteit van Amsterdam.

Chapter 6

The Phonetic / Phonologic Program

As speech therapists will verify, the phonetic/phonologic area is sometimes presented as the "simple" area of practice. Articulation disorders are often the first problems upon which the student of speech pathology is allowed to vent all her newly acquired zeal and prowess; they are supposed to be the least of our problems! However, when we look at the many differing approaches to the remediation of articulatory disorders, or when we stop to ask ourselves what articulation is, we find that the subject is far from simple. The clinician can ascertain fairly easily that the child is suffering from a disorder of articulation, but she then has to identify the probable cause of the disorder. Is the child suffering from auditory-processing disorders or does he have a neuromuscular deficit? Maybe the problem is psychogenic, as described by Myklebust (1960). In our diagnostic sessions we may use standardized tests, informal sampling, or distinctive feature analysis, as described by Menyuk (1968). We may subscribe to the Van Riper (1972) approach, a motokinesthetic approach, as outlined by Young and Hawk (1965), or a multiphonemic approach; but whatever the cause or prognosis, many clinicians tackle articulation disorders in a personal and sometimes rigid manner. Seldom are the mother's modeling and corrective practices monitored and modified, and yet, frequently, faulty articulation (for whatever cause) produces anxiety and inappropriate corrective practices in the mother. Furthermore, articulation therapy is often supported by "homework" schedules, and yet little is done to ensure that the interactive interchanges between mother and child will allow for learning to take place.

It has certainly not been attempted, within the confines of this text, to present a treatise on articulation disorders, but rather it is intended that such disorders be discussed within the framework of our original graphic model (see Chapter 1). The hypothesis is again that using the mother as an agent of therapy ensures that her "clinical" practices will be modified and that the child will therefore benefit from more normal interactions in the home.

For the purposes of discussion, articulation disorders are divided into three catagories: linguistic problems, motokinesthetic problems, and/or behavioral problems. "Linguistic problems" is used as a global term that covers all children who are unable to handle the phonetic/phonologic element of their basic grammar, as described by Chomsky (1957), for the many and varied reasons that are more commonly referred to as "processing problems." The term motokinesthetic problems covers the children who suffer from neurologically based deficits of motokinesthetic origin. Finally, the "behavioral problems" includes those who suffer from neither of the former deficits, but who nevertheless display articulation errors. As Pollack and Rees (1972) have indicated, it is important to make these distinctions, for one child may have a phonetic disorder while the other suffers from a phonemic disorder. Pollack and Rees (1972) described the child who suffers from the phonetic problem as having anomalies of the orofacial area, sequencing difficulties, or neurological disorders that produce incorrect articulation even though the child may have acquired an adult system of phonologic rules. These children have the characteristics of the "neurologically based deficit." Pollack and Rees (1972) then describe the child with the phonemic disorder as one who uses his own phonemic rules. These children could have linguistic deficits but it is possible that behavioral problems also contribute to their disorder.

Whichever group we are dealing with, we have some grave and fundamental problems to tackle, particularly in light of our foregoing discussions.

First, if we subscribe to Sussman's (1972) theories concerning "what the tongue tells the brain," in which he describes a closed-loop feedback system by which the tongue supplies the central nervous system with information about spatial orientation, direction, and velocity, or articulatory movement, then we agree that incorrect articulation can only be an incorrect reinforcer. If this is the case, then all of our children suffering from articulation disorders are reinforcing their own incorrect patterns. Conversely, both Dale (1976) and Ling (1976) have indicated that corrections of misarticulations may inhibit and restrict the flow of language and its creation. Ling (1976) outlines in minute detail the importance of all sense modalities in speech production and states that correct patterns of coarticulation are of paramount importance both to the "feedback" and "feed forward" systems of articulation.

Inherent in these arguments is what seems to be an insoluble problem: the protagonists on the one side are claiming that faulty articulation must be corrected, and the antagonists on the other side are claiming that corrective practices are dangerous to language learning. We also have to remenber that faulty articulation can lead to critically damaging corrective practices on the part of the anxious, nagging parent.

The ideal therapy, therefore, would be one that incorporates parental guidance and support and that is built around realistic goals and expectations. Correct reinforcement schedules should again be developed, and every effort should be made to ensure that all parental modeling is correct as far as phonology is concerned. Second, corrective practices of the phonetic/phonologic element of language should not be allowed to interfere with the child's experiments with the semantic and syntactic elements. Last, the mother-clinician should follow a corrective procedure that helps eliminate the dangers inherent in Sussman's (1972) theories.

To this end, this clinician believes that there can be no more suitable practice than that outlined by Ling (1976). He described an approach to coarticulation that is built on a mastery of subskills to produce a target behavior. He suggested that speech skills can be improved if drill sessions with careful selective reinforcement schedules are practiced two or three times daily with the clinician or an informed parent. He compared this to the child's own drill sessions. Ling (1976) suggests that phonetic drill allows for corrective practices without being restrictive to language flow; thus he avoids the problems foreseen by Dale (1976). Before the implementation of the drill sessions, the manner, place, and voicing of all sounds in spontaneous speech is assessed. Remediation is then geared to a specific set of subskills for a target coarticulated production. Ling (1976) discussed in his book the teaching of all subskills from plain voicing to intricate, coarticulated triple consonant blends in a vowel environment, and claims that systematic teaching and evaluation is the optimum route to success. He advised that phonetic competence is gained through drill procedures, but that phonologic skill will be achieved only through the child's constant experience of correct linguistic interchanges. Hence, there is an overlap with the language procedures already described.

Perhaps it is now appropriate to discuss how these theories, as outlined and practiced by Ling (1976), and our own subsequent adaptation of them "fit" with some of the better known theories of articulation, diagnosis, and remediation.

Winitz (1969) pointed out that, in building improved articulatory behaviors, competition between new and old responses is important and that correction of the old responses should be minimal. Van Riper (1972) also suggested that a new pattern of movement has to be learned and new goals set. Both of these views would be adhered to in the implementation of Ling's (1976) theories concerning reinforcement practices. Carrier (1970) discussed using a target sound and precise reinforcement practices, and Griffiths and Craighead (1972) found that reinforcement did appear to facilitate therapy. In the ensuing program, correct selective and motivational reinforcement schedules are of paramount importance. Finally, the idea of using the mother as an agent of therapy has been discussed by both Carrier (1970) and Morley and Fox (1967). The former has shown how his program for parents accelerates the generalization of clinically elicited practices and minimizes the use of the clinician's time. Morley and Fox (1969) point out that the child spends the greater part of his early life with his mother, who may have become over anxious about the disordered articulation. They suggest that this anxiety might best be allayed if the mother is shown ways in which she can help. The suggestion in this text that new target behaviors should be carefully goaled, specifically and positively reinforced, and presented for implementation, is far from being new, and should be acceptable from many theoretical points of view.

The following phonetic drill chart is presented as an adaptation of all such procedures and for use when and where a child's articulation patterns indicate. The individual clinician will have no difficulty in modifying the program for her own, her patient's or the clinical mother's needs. Obviously, careful diagnosis must be carried out to determine which part of the articulatory program should be used. Again, the outline included here is adapted for the mother's appreciation, understanding, and use, and therefore international phonetic symbols are discarded in favor of standard spelling. Prosodic skills can and should also be incorporated by varying the pitch, rhythm, and stress of the articulated sequences. As yet, research has not indicated a developmental hierarchy of prosodic features. Brown (1977) does, however, cite six prosodic features of the mother's speech as isolated by Garnica, which are:

1. A higher fundamental frequency
2. A greater pitch range
3. A rising terminal frequency

4. Occasional whispering
5. Longer duration in speaking separable verbs, e.g., *go out.*
6. Two primary syllabic stresses on words calling for one.

Furthermore, Crystal (1973) pointed out that the organizing of intonation into segmented chunks is a grammatical function that appears very early in the infant's life. He suggests that prosodic features are even present in the birth cry. At this stage of research, therefore, it is vital that the importance of prosody be recognized. Because of the lack of empirical developmental data, it is suggested that prosodic features should be superimposed once a child has mastered manner, place, and voicing of the target coarticulated sound.

SOUND TEACHING CHART

Vowels: Practice quick repetitions of the underlined sounds and check the appropriate column when the child can:

(a)   Copy them quickly
(b)   Vary the pitch and rhythm
(c)   Use them in spontaneous speech

	a	b	c
cart			
bean			
moon			
fork			
day			
girl			
house			
boy			
hat			
pin			
egg			
hot			
cup			

Alternate the above sounds quickly.
NOTE: Use no more than a minute or two for each drill session. Remember: 'Fun' activity as reward.

Consonants: Check (a), (b), and (c) as before. Use with vowels as directed (v = vowels).

Lips	a	b	c	Tongue Front	a	b	c	Tongue Back	a	b	c
w before v's				t before or after v's				k before or after v's			
p before or after v's				d before or after v's				g before or after v's			
b before or after v's				n before or after v's				ng after v's			
m before or after v's				s before or after v's				h before v's			
f before or after v's				z before or after v's							
v before or after v's				ch before or after v's							
Mix any two of the above.				sh before or after v's							
				j before or after v's							
				l before v's							
				r before v's							
				Mix any two of the above.							

More than one consonant at the beginning:

Lips	a	b	c	Tongue Front	a	b	c	Tongue Back	a	b	c
sm before v				fl before v				kr before v			
sp before v				fr before v				tr before v			
sw before v				pr before v				skr before v			
sl before v				tw before v				spr before v			
sn before v				kw(qu) before v				skw(squ) before v			
bl before v				dr before v				str before v			
pl before v				gl before v							
br before v											

More than one consonant at the end (*words are for examples*):

	a	b	c		a	b	c
lm—film				gl—giggle			
ln—kiln				gz—pigs			
lz—balls				kl—tickle			
mz—arms				ks—knocks			
nz—buns				ps—pops			
vz—gloves				tl—little			
ft—soft				kt—kicked			
ld—old				pt—hopped			
lp—gulp				gd—begged			
lt—belt				bd—rubbed			
mp—jump							
nd—hand				fts—lifts			
nt—bent				kts—acts			
ngk—junk				mblz—mumbles			
sk—whisk				mpl—simple			
sp—wasp							
vd—dived				skt—asked			
pl—topple				spt—lisped			
bl—table				ndz—stands			
bz—tubs				nts—points			
dl—cradle				ngkl—ankle			
dz—beads							
tn—kitten							

NOTE: No more than a minute or two—*Fun, please.*

TEACHING THE DRILL

The format for the "drill sessions" incorporating the above program can be described briefly. The mother and child work toward an articulatory achievement, but a reinforcing play activity is used when the goal is achieved. The therapist demonstrates to the mother how to say one of the "sounds" outlined in the above chart, the child repeats it, and, if he is correct, he is allowed to carry out some performance task, e.g., place a puzzle piece. The child is also positively reinforced verbally. Care should be taken to use very precise reinforcement techniques, and the mother should be closely observed in relation to this. If the child's efforts are incorrect, a comment such as "That was a good try," rather than "No, that was wrong" is more motivationally reinforcing, which is of great import in the light of the ideas propounded in previous chapters. However, a "Yes, put a piece in" to an incorrect utterance would obviously be a dangerous teaching practice. It is vital, therefore, that the mother's reinforcement practices be monitored in detail.

This clinician has found that the reinforcement practices and activities are invaluable and that in her experience the great majority of children love these drill sessions. Care should be taken, however, not to extend the drill sessions beyond Ling's (1976) recommended two or three minutes twice or thrice daily. The child's evident enjoyment seems to suggest that here again Ling (1976) has outlined an extremely valuable therapeutic procedure for the diagnosis, evaluation, and remediation of articulatory skills.

SUMMARY

This chapter has presented a phonetic program for the mother's use with her articulation-disordered child. The novel format of the program and its implementation do not defy, but rather encompass, many traditional theories on articulation and its remediation. Specific attention is given to prosody as well as to manner, place, and voicing, and reinforcement is seen as an important variable.

REFERENCES

Brown, R. 1977. The place of baby talk in the world of language. In: C. Snow and C. Ferguson (eds.), Talking to Children. Cambridge University Press, New York.

Carrier, A. 1970. A program of articulation therapy administered by mothers. JSHD 35(4):344–353.

Chomsky, N. 1957. Syntactic Structures. Mouton, The Hague.

Crystal, D. 1973. Linguistic mythology and the first year of life. Br. J. Dis. Comm. 8(1):29–36.

Dale, P. S. 1976. Language Development: Structure and Function, 2nd Ed. Holt, Rinehart & Winston, New York.

Griffiths, H., and W. E. Craighead. 1972. Generalization in operant speech therapy for misarticulation. JSHD 37(4):485–494.

Ling, D. 1976. Speech and the Hearing-Impaired child: Theory and Practice. The Alexander Graham Bell Association for the Deaf, Washington, D.C.

Menyuk, P. 1968. The role of distinctive features in children's acquisition of phonology. JSHR 11:138–146 March.

Morley, M. and J. Fox. 1969. Disorders of articulation, theory and therapy. BJDC 4(2):151–165.

Myklebust, H. R. 1960. The Psychology of Deafness. Grune & Stratton, New York.

Pollack, E., and N. Rees. 1972. Disorders of articulation. Some clinical implications of distinctive feature therapy. JSHD 37(4): 451–461.

Sussman, H. 1972. What the tongue tells the brain. Psychol. Bull. 77(4):262–272 April.

Van Riper, C. 1972. Speech Correction Principles and Methods. Constable & Co., London.

Winitz, H. 1969. Articulation, Acquisition and Behavior. Appleton-Century-Crofts, New York.

Young, E., and S. Hawk. 1965. Motor-Kinaesthetic Speech Training. Stanford University Press, Stanford, California.

PART 2

APPLICATION OF THE CLINICAL PRACTICE TO PARTICULAR HEARING-, LANGUAGE-, AND SPEECH-DISORDERED POPULATIONS

Introduction

The second part of this text applies the theories and practices already discussed to particular children and particular situations. Included are suggestions for using these theories in the treatment of specific disorders, for example, mental retardation or hearing impairment. There are also case histories with discussions in which this writer gives some subjective opinions about how applications of these theories have helped, or might help, in overcoming the problems presented. An apology is made for the general nature of the overview. Many of the children discussed were treated by this clinician before her ideas were formulated quite as they are presented herein, but the basic principles were the same. At the time that much of the treatment described here was underway, data were being collected only to facilitate the optimum treatment of the child in question. "Scientific methodology" was not always adhered to. This clinician has learned all too late that there are many reasons for keeping systematic data other than for treatment of the clinical child! The discussion ahead, therefore, does not include data resulting from scientific clinical research; the information must be understood to be what it is, i.e., observed data discussed in a highly subjective manner. It is easy to make excuses on the grounds of clinical pressures, particularly as a lone clinician working in a vast, semi-industrial, semi-rural area, in a country as large as Australia, with as few speech pathologists as it has; the temptation is always to see and to treat the next patient rather than to keep clinical records in proper research fashion. The pressures of the waiting list and the anxious angry voice on the telephone are always there: "When will you see my child, we've been waiting a year?" This writer, therefore, had to decide whether to include in the following discussion a few case histories with clinical research presentations, or a variety of material that has been collected, observed, and recorded over a span of twenty years. The second course was chosen for a number of reasons. First, some of the children, parents, and interactions discussed are rare examples of a type of behavior. Second, it can be argued that, however precise clinical methods become, the clinician must use subjectivity in her decisions and in her observations; it is a variable that can never be excluded, nor should it be. Finally, there is a plea herein to all clinicians to compile and to pass on as much available data as possible. It is the author's belief that the most humble of clinics has as much to offer the researchers in their own discipline as the researchers have to contribute to the practice of speech pathology.

Part 2 is therefore mainly a clinical discussion, the greatest portion of which is devoted to the hearing-impaired child. Again, the emphasis given to this disorder is highly subjective; it is the predominant field in which the writer is currently working. It is also a field in which, the writer believes, the "whole chain of circumstances we call communication has broken down"; not because of the hearing impairment, but rather because of the other variables to which this text is devoted. It could be that the other disorders discussed deserve more attention than they receive; that is for specialists in those fields to consider.

Chapter 7
Application to the
Partially Hearing Child

One of the most enlightening of this writer's earliest professional experiences was working with two young teachers of the deaf who were fighting the tide of tradition. They believed simply in the use of residual hearing and parental guidance in the management of young partially hearing children at least in the initial stages and whatever the degree of loss. Their results had a profound effect upon this clinician. The teachers' names were Daniel and Agnes Ling. Since those days, the Lings have done much, through their research, writing, and teaching, to qualify their ideas. However, despite their findings, and those of others such as Wedenberg (1951), Whetnall and Fry (1971), Pollack and Rees (1972), and Goldstein (1939), to name only a few, there has been an alarming reversal to total communication and to visually dominant methods of teaching the hearing-impaired child. Cued speech, as outlined by Cornett (1967), is just one example of a visually based system that has been developed in the past decades.

In the light of recent research findings, which are discussed later, and also because of the ideas already outlined in this text, the writer finds this reversal abhorrent and herein presents a hypothetical model to substantiate her arguments.

DISCUSSION OF
GRAPHIC MODEL FOR THE USE OF AUDITION

The Graphic Model is a hypothetical diagram presented in an attempt to conceptualize the need for linguistic input, leaving the visual and kinesthetic modalities for the cognitive and extraverbal cues so critical to language learning. Study of Figure 7.1 will show two children presented in diagrammatic form, one representing the hearing child and the other representing the partially hearing child. Between the two are listed the elements of language as presented by current linguistic and psycholinguistic doctrine. We must ask ourselves how this language is presented to the child, through which sensory modalities it passes, how it is received and stored in the brain, and how it is transformed into expressive speech and language.

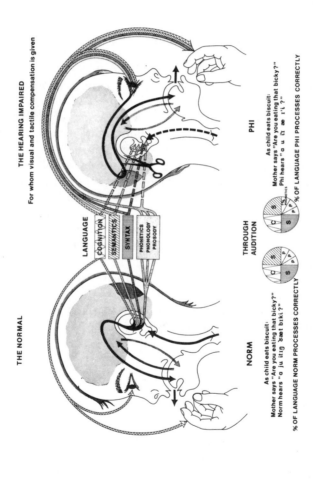

Figure 7.1.   Hypothetical model of dominant modalities of language speech chain for NORM (Normally hearing child) and PHI (Partially hearing child to whom visual and tactile compensation is given).

What are the contrasts in the processes that cause a difference between the utterances of the normal child and those of the hearing-impaired child? As this is a *hypothetical* discussion let us leave the level of hearing for later analysis. To cause visual dominance as is indicated in the diagram, the child must have a loss severe enough to make the acquisition of normal language an "impossibility" (Silverman and Davis, 1970). The underlying transcribed message, in the model, "Are you eating that bicky?" should provide a comparative basis for discussion.

The most obvious contrast between the two children in the model is that one is drawn with the left hemisphere of the brain showing and the other with the right hemisphere showing. This is not without a reason, which will shortly be presented. Second, the modalities through which the elements of language reach the brain differ dramatically. Let us discuss this in detail; in so doing we accept that the child needs to perceive and learn the 1) cognitive, 2) semantic, 3) syntactic, and 4) P/P/P (phonetic, phonologic, and prosodic) elements of his language.

The child on our left is the hackneyed Normal. The child on our right is PHI (partially hearing impaired). PHI is diagnosed as having a hearing loss, and either by design or by accident compensatory measures are immediately introduced. It could be that a child is fitted with an aid under the assumption that he will use his residual hearing, but this is not that easy for him. He and his teachers, his parents, his clinician, his siblings, and his peers, all want to quickly compensate him for his terrible handicap. What happens to the ingoing language elements? We will study each in its turn.

COGNITION (Figure 7.2)   (Understanding of Extraverbal Stimuli)

NORM   learns through all modalities, i.e., audition, vision, and kinesthetic (represented graphically by the hand).

PHI   does much the same, but the auditory input is "cut" (see scissors in Figure 7.1).

SEMANTICS (Figure 7.3)   (The Label, Symbol, Word, or Meaning for What He Has Perceived and Understood)

NORM   learns through audition dominantly, and matches what he learns to a visual cue.

PHI   learns through vision and/or touch (written word, lip reading, gestures and signs, or finger spelling, and maybe concurrent impaired audition).
It goes without saying that he will favor the easiest modality. Immediacy is important to the child.

SYNTAX (Figure 7.4)   (Grammar or rules from which to create the endless computations that result in creative speech)

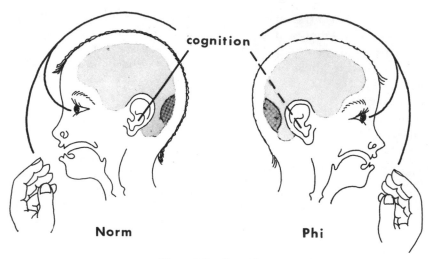

Figure 7.2.   Cognition.

NORM   Receives these dominantly through audition, which he links to extraverbal cues.

PHI   Again receives these through vision and/or touch with a smattering of audition.

P/P/P (Figure 7.5)   (Phonetics—sounds; Phonology—meanings attached to these sounds; Prosody—stress, pitch, rhythm, length, pauses)

NORM   receives all 3 P's through audition again.

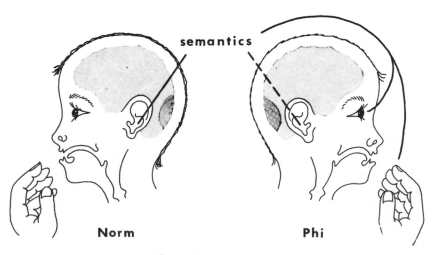

Figure 7.3.   Semantics.

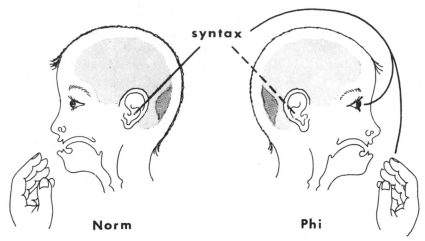

Figure 7.4. Syntax.

PHI   receives all 3 P's predominantly through vision and/or kinesthetic
        modality.

Note that the modalities are not mentioned exclusively, but
rather the arguments concern reception of the ingoing data through
the dominant modalities. The next stage is to hypothesize what happens to the information after reception; in other words, where does it
go in the brain, and how does the brain use it?

Obviously, it is impossible to present empirical data, for as Luria
(1976) said, "There is an extreme shortage of reliable evidence

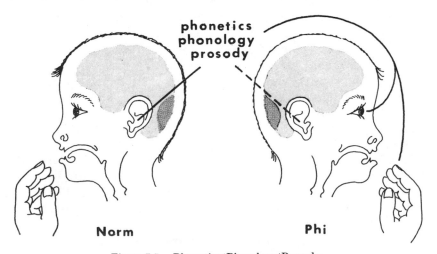

Figure 7.5. Phonetics/Phonology/Prosody.

regarding the nondominant hemisphere." However, he goes on to state categorically that the right hemisphere plays no part in the organization of speech and language activity. Lesions of the left hemisphere are what produce speech and language deficits in patients. We can therefore assume that the data collected by NORM will be processed predominantly, but not necessarily exclusively, in the language centers of the left hemisphere. As already explained, the linguistic input is mostly bound within the auditory modality. For this reason, our figure shows the linguistic information passing from NORM's ears up to the left hemisphere of his brain. The diagram of PHI, however, shows data passing from the eye (or visual modality) to the right hemisphere of the brain, which Luria said plays no part in the organization of speech. He does state that lesions of the right hemisphere cause disturbances of visual perception. Kimura (1963) found that such lesions also lead to the disturbance of the ability to recognize objects, and Luria finally suggested that they produce a disturbance of the body schema and spatial disorientation. This information suggests that a great deal of the data carried by the visual modality are processed in the right hemisphere, which substantiates Owrid's (1977) arguments in his discussions of Trevoort's findings—that a visual system of language is predominantly spatial and not time based. Owrid claimed that visual communicators, i.e., PHI, are predominantly concerned with spatial properties that are concrete, as opposed to audiologic communicators, i.e., NORM, whose language, is metaphorical and time based. Similarly, Ivimey (1976) stated that the language of the deaf child, while having its own rules, is predominantly external (this could be interpreted as spatial and concrete) while the language of the normal child is internalized (through left hemisphere processing).

There is some evidence from neurologic findings that information from the auditory modality will reach the left hemisphere predominantly, while information from the visual modality will be processed in the right hemisphere predominantly; hence the graphic representations of NORM and PHI. The contrast appears to be marked and suggests that PHI has (at least graphically) a heavily overloaded visual system. It was Ling (1976) who discussed the disadvantages of such overloading in terms of both short-term and long-term memory capacity. He raised doubts about the ability of the child to process such a vast quantity of data through one modality, while still leaving that modality free to function as it was intended, i.e., for the processing of cognitive and extraverbal data.

Further comparative study of NORM and PHI shows that the processing differences do not end even at this stage, but are continued with the expressive elements of language. In NORM's case the linguistic data are passed from the left hemisphere to the producers of outgoing speech. As Sussman (1972) said, the tongue then feeds back to the brain all the articulatory information. Ling (1976) discussed the ensuing feed-forward mechanisms that produce ongoing articulatory skills.

PHI, in contrast, will receive predominantly visual information, rather than acoustic and linguistic information, which will then be fed forward into the expressive system. His articulation is consequently at risk, and incorrect patterns are fed back to the brain, where they reinforce incorrect learning and feed forward incorrect articulatory practices. The reaction of this clinician is "poor, poor, PHI," and all this is done because he is said to be unable to hear. Is he allowed to process what he does hear through the proper linguistic and neurologic channels, or is he at risk despite his hearing? It is this clinician's belief that he is primarily at risk because of what we do to him, or at best, because of what happens to him, rather than because of his hearing loss. It could even be that by using such modality imbalance and upsetting the innate processing capacities of the child, we are introducing dysphasic qualities or retrocochlear lesions. Much audiologic research is currently geared to differential diagnosis of central as opposed to cochlear lesions, yet in older children these could well be acquired because of misguided communication stratagems. Dysphasia is a rare condition in childhood, but it appears that dysphasic qualities can indeed be taught. There are many who hear but cannot interpret what they hear because they have been inadequately taught; the assumption was made that they could not hear and that they could communicate only through visual compensation.

Let us take this argument further and ask ourselves just what the child needs to hear. We note from our model that both NORM and PHI are eating a biscuit in the company of their mothers, and the mother says:

> "Are you eating that bicky?"
> NORM hears: "ɑ̃ ju itɪŋ ðæt bɪki?"
> PHI hears: "ɑ u iʼɪ æ ɪ̆ʼi"

Which of the basic elements of the message (as shown in Figures 7.2–7.5) are carried to each child? What of the cognitive, semantic, syntactic, and P/P/P elements; who could receive which elements if audition alone were used for both children?

COGNITIVE   NORM and PHI both receive this element; they know what they are doing.

SEMANTIC   Both can process this element through audition because they know that what they hear must be matched to the extra-verbal cues.

SYNTACTIC   NORM and PHI can both construct a distinctive grammar from what they hear. To PHI, "Are you eating that bicky?" (ɑ̈ ju itɪŋ ðæt bɪki?) will sound different from, "Will you eat that bicky!" (ɪ 'ʊ ju i æ ɪ'i). Stress intonation and vowel format are all different.

P/P/P   NORM will hear the phonetic element—all the sounds. He can use these for the phonologic element. He will also hear all the prosodic features. PHI will not hear all the phonetic element, but will certainly hear a large percentage, even if he is profoundly deaf. He can use what he hears phonologically. Much of the stress, pitch, rhythm, and intonation will be heard. It must be remembered that audiograms cannot show duration of sound, and much of the prosodic element of language is carried through just this feature.

If, therefore, we compare the pi diagrams in Figure 7.1, we will see that there is little difference between the two hypothetical children's abilities to process all the known elements of language through audition. The minimal percentage difference shows that only the phonetic element is at risk inherently. Compensatory tactics have, however, caused all elements—with the possible exception of the cognitive—to be at risk.

Northern and Downs (1974) have stated that there is little reason to be proud of educational attainments in the management of the hearing-impaired child. They cite these main reasons:

1. An inability to accept change
2. An inability to recognize the educational implications of modern research
3. A lack of research and castigation on the part of those who depart from traditional approaches
4. An overwhelming desire to maintain the status quo

It is this clinician's belief that the current linguistic and neurologic information, along with the acoustic data presented by Ling (1976), can no longer be ignored. It must be utilized if the hearing-impaired child is to receive optimum help. We must add that all other variables mentioned earlier in this text have to be considered: the mother, the environment, the reinforcement channels, and the anxiety levels. What happens to these in relation to the hearing-impaired child? We have studied PHI himself, and also his linguistic input, but what does he do to his environment, and how do his interchanges compare with NORM's? A discussion of each of the variables mentioned above follows.

PHI'S MOTHER, HER ANXIETY LEVELS, HER REINFORCEMENT SCHEDULES, AND HER LINGUISTIC PRACTICES

As mentioned in earlier chapters, it would be appropriate to try to identify and modify anxiety-based behaviors before initiating a therapeutic program. It is not too difficult to accept that PHI's mother, or the mother of any child diagnosed as having a hearing loss, will be prey to anxiety. We must establish at what level she experiences this anxiety; for if it reaches a neurotic level then she will be unable to react appropriately to her child's stimuli. It is critical for the clinician to realize just how many factors could produce anxiety in the mother, and to realize that each new anxiety stimulus may have to be tackled independently through diagnosis and counseling. Some of the many anxiety-producing situations and the possible resultant behaviors are discussed below.

Initial Diagnosis

PHI's mother will be anxious (undoubtedly beyond the normal level) about the initial diagnostic visits, whether they be to the general practitioner, consultant, or audiologist. This anxiety will probably be generalized throughout the family, to relations, and to friends. We remind ourselves that such anxiety produces anger, criticism, lack of love, and lack of communication, so that just when PHI needs the full support of his mother he may find himself facing the investigatory onslaught of headphones, probes, hospital gowns, noises, crowds, separation, and confusion with a mother who suddenly becomes angry and hostile. Many clinicians will have seen this symptomatic behavior acted out daily in the waiting room. This may continue for a long period of time, in many different situations, and with many different people. Furthermore, as the diagnosis of a hearing loss becomes more and more inevitable, PHI's mother's anxiety will lead to a change in her behavior at home. Her preconceived construct of what deafness "is" will also induce altered attitudes. Because of her anxiety she will talk and play less, but also she will begin to feel that it is useless to talk because "he can't hear." PHI will withdraw and lack motivation, he will possibly become negative toward his mother, his babble or chatter will reduce, and, therefore, his mother will not be reinforced—except in the belief that deaf children are mute. Thus, the mutually reinforcing state of anxiety increases. The clinician who is able to help at this stage is indeed most fortunate. Play sessions should be monitored, and modification should take place according to the overt behaviors that are present. Above all, the parents should be counseled, they should be informed of what is happening, and why they feel as they do. If they can accept that their feelings of anxiety are normal but that it is these very feelings that are producing the negative symptoms on either side, they will readily modify these feelings and begin to advance. Likewise, even before diagnosis is made, the preconceived ideas about what deafness "is" must be supplanted by thoughts of what can be done for the child with partial hearing.

The Hearing Aids

The aids are another anxiety-producing stimulus. Even the normally anxious mother must wonder where to get them, how to fit them, how to work them, how not to break them, and what other people will think of them. PHI's mother will be superhuman if her anxiety about these matters does not affect her behavior toward PHI. For example, he may run toward the sea, which he has finally decided he likes because of his mother's patient and loving encouragement, but now she shouts at him angrily to keep away. (He will ruin his hearing aid). He may go to talk to the neighbor and find that he is stopped. (His mother is frightened of the reaction to the hearing aid.) His "ears" may be taken on and off in a most confusing manner, and he may come to hate this delightful noise producer because it is a source of so much anger and attention from his mother. If it goes wrong, he will be blamed for pouring milk into it, tripping over it, standing on it, or fiddling with it; in many cases it will be the first time that money values are thrown at him in anxious, threatening terminology.

The intelligent mother will also have begun reading about the subject, and she will become anxious about and threatened by the type of aids available and the choice of the type most suited to PHI's loss. Unless she is counseled about the audiogram, its meaning, its advantages, its shortcomings, and the type of aid fitted, her anxiety will only increase. She may think of the aid in terms of cosmetic rather than linguistic-acoustic variables. She may think of the aid in terms of the listener (PHI) rather than the speaker (herself), when both, in fact, should receive her consideration. She may think of the aid in terms of financial deficit. All this must be sensibly evaluated at a level of normal anxiety and must be channeled into a constructive response and a positive or productive outcome for herself, the family, and, above all, her partially hearing child.

Developmental Milestones

There are few diagnoses of a sensorineural loss that are not associated with "risk factors," and most mothers are aware that "risk factors" can produce a multiplicity of deficits. It is therefore almost inevitable that the mother of PHI will be profoundly anxious about numerous symptoms that she feels may be looming on the horizon. She will watch his development, in all probability neurotically rather than with pleasure, and if he is late with the cutting of a tooth, in her mind it will be a disaster. Inevitably her behavior toward PHI will be affected. Analysis of mother's speech at this stage may well show a reduction in Brown's (1977) affection content, and an imbalance in the type of statements made. There will, probably be many more imperative statements than is the norm. PHI's mother will be pushing him to reach all those milestones that she fears so dreadfully he will miss, because she imagines multiple deficits. At best, she may fear that his hearing loss will produce a global deficiency. Of course, it will be this very fear and her resultant behaviors that produce such a deficit rather than the hearing loss itself. Yet, the latter will inevitably be blamed for all the ills, not only by the mother but by many of the personnel with whom she comes into contact. It is therefore reiterated that unless PHI is treated within the parameters suggested by our original Model (Figure 1.1) it will be impossible to assess and modify all the factors that should receive the clinician's attention. The more we think about it the more it becomes apparent that PHI's hearing loss and possible language deficit are only a small cog in a bewildering chain of events. Again, however, an awareness of, counseling for, and, finally, a modification of overt behaviors through the methods outlined in Chapter 2 can do much to prevent this chain of events from occurring.

The Mother's Own Capabilities

In the current climate of childhood analysis and psychiatric opinion on optimal parental management, there can be few parents who do not, at some time, doubt their own capabilities in childhood management. Many parents have doubts that reach a neurotic level, even if their children have no apparent clinical problem. Therefore, PHI's parents are again at an immediate disadvantage. It is unlikely that they have ever experienced partial hearing at close quarters, and they will inevitably see the task ahead of them as a tremendous burden to which they are hopelessly and inadequately suited. The problem may seem so enormous that they will elect to give up and hand over PHI lock, stock, and barrel to "them," i.e., the State authorities in charge of deafness. Whichever path they choose, the results can hardly be beneficial to PHI unless his parents are given adequate counseling, guidance, and support. If, in the first instance, the parents are left to fend for themselves with only the barest of counseling services, they will almost inevitably adopt many of the anxiety-based behaviors already discussed, to say nothing of the linguistic practices induced by PHI's lack of response. Conversely, if they hand PHI over to the State system, he will never receive the healthy, cognitive, emotional, and linguistic environments so necessary for his optimum development. If the parents can be involved in the therapeutic program, they can begin to conceptualize their own and their child's efforts in a manner that can produce a happy, healthy interchange for all concerned.

Preconceived Ideas of Deafness

Intelligence, marriage, schooling, career, and appearance: all these will bring doubts and anxieties to PHI's parents. Again, the anxieties identified will result in damaging behaviors. All the constructs that the parents may have must, of course, be discussed in counseling, but counseling about and discussion of the phenomena that are worrying the parents are not enough if the child is to be treated within the framework of his total environment. Interactive schedules must be assessed and treated, where necessary.

Language and Speech

Language and speech are the areas about which even the most ill-informed of parents will have the most anxiety. We all know that deaf people cannot talk, or so it is still believed by a vast majority of the populace. How will these misconceptions affect the mother-child reinforcement schedules and linguistic interchanges? The mother will have strong preconceived ideas about what compensatory measures she should take; she will have seen deaf-mutes gesturing; she will have seen emotive films on the subject; and, above all, she will have highly personalized ideas about what speech and language are and how she could best elicit both understanding and expression from her child.

Probably the most obvious and most common feature of the mother-child linguistic interchange involving a nonverbal child is the heavy reliance upon gesture. This is particularly apparent with the partially hearing child, and it is this clinician's experience that the gesturing of PHI's mother will be far more situationally encompassing than the deixis described by Newport et al. (1977) as being so important in the normal mother-child interchange. It is possible to elaborate on this point. In the case of NORM, the mother, on explaining to her child that she wishes him to feed himself, for example, initially shows him plate, spoon, and the movement of the spoon in the required manner. This could be termed deixis, and may be accompanied by such words as "Come on darling, you try and feed yourself." NORM would match the words with the extraverbal cues, and his resulting performance would reinforce his mother to the effect that he has understood. The deixis would not be needed again to such an extent and would therefore gradually be reduced, but the linguistic utterance would be maintained, expanded, and adopted on future occasions. The linguistic input therefore becomes the predominant one. In PHI's case a similar routine may be enacted, and his mother will likewise receive reinforcement that he has "understood." However, even if she utters a full sentence (in many cases unlikely), she is still prone to the belief that he cannot hear the utterance, and so she goes on using the elaborate deixis as her prime means of communication. The linguistic input may be reduced or may be discarded in favor of continuing the mime, which is elaborated and expanded upon just as the linguistic material was in the case of NORM. The child's nonverbal reply to his mother's example only reinforces her belief in his mutism, and so a punishing interaction is introduced, at least for language learning.

Despite this, it is not suggested that the mother becomes completely silent, but it is apparent to this clinician that PHI's mother almost invariably becomes a "clinical" mother at least in her linguistic interchanges. Let us elaborate on this, and in so doing discuss the earliest levels of language competence as outlined in Chapters 4 and 5.

In the case of NORM, during the concrete stage of his development, when mother is busy providing nouns and noun-phrase structures, she is able to see from NORM's actions that he has understood her. Occasionally, he will reinforce her with his own utterance, but she receives her reinforcement and her cues both from what he is doing and from what he is saying. She does not insist on direct imitation from the child before she provides more linguistic data; she is confident in her interchange. In PHI's case, however, the mother has a preconceived idea that he will not understand and that only when he has said a word can he possibly know it. Consequently, a great deal of time is spent in encouraging PHI to say "doggy," for only when he has said "doggy" will the mother really believe that he knows the word "doggy"! Her teaching practices deviate from the normal (as discussed in Chapter 4) dramatically. Teaching frequently becomes imitative rather than interactive, with all the inherent dangers already mentioned. Input is reduced until the mother is reinforced by her child's utterance. (We must ask ourselves if such practices result from the mother's example alone, or could they apply to the formal teaching as well?) Perhaps most dangerous of all, the mother does not cue in from her child's cognitive explorations, but persists with just two or three words that she feels will mean the pinnacle of success if only she can persuade PHI to utter them. This constant and sustained effort will soon cause a "plateauing" of the child's language at a concrete level. There are so many nouns a child must learn—all the names of all objects—that the language becomes persistently concrete at the expense of generative transformational syntactic principles. Even when the child does repeat the required noun, it is unlikely to be expanded and modified as it would be in a healthy interchange. A more probable request to PHI would be "You said it! He said 'doggy.' Say it again. Show Mummy (Daddy, Granny, and Mrs. Jones) you can say 'doggy'." All this is said, regardless of whether or not the child is interested, and whether or not there is a doggy in view. What of the expansion into "the big black furry dog who is jumping"? That would appear to be lost forever.

It is not suggested that verb phrases are never used with PHI, for indeed they are, but again the interchange becomes stifling. Lack of interaction and expansion prohibits normal linguistic experimenting. If only the child were allowed to experiment, he might develop some skills on his own despite a profound hearing loss.

For a final comparison between NORM's and PHI's linguistic experiences, let us discuss what happens to NORM if he does not understand his mother's utterance (and there are numerous occasions on which this will happen before he will achieve full linguistic competence). The mother will probably see that NORM does not understand, and she will automatically expand or rephrase her utterance—maybe with added deixis— to encompass data that she is sure he knows and that will help him to understand. NORM will busily process what he hears, match it to the situational cues, and then respond, he hopes, appropriately. The experiment will be repeated until success is realized, but all the time the linguistic input will be adapted toward his understanding. NORM begins to use the linguistic data to achieve the required level of understanding, and, in so doing, must inevitably advance his processing abilities.

In PHI's case, a lack of understanding will produce a totally different response from the person with whom he is interacting. PHI's mother, for example, will immediately assume that he has not heard, cannot hear, and therefore will never understand the linguistic input, so she compensates in any way she thinks fit. Usually, this encompasses advanced gesturing, changed behavioral attitudes, and severely reduced utterances—often to the level of one word—which in itself reduces the syntactic message carried in the utterance. PHI is not given the opportunity to experiment linguistically; it is immediately denied him. If, however, he were able to hear the difficult utterance more frequently than NORM does and if he were allowed to process the data and to link it with the extraverbal cues just as NORM does, he would surely understand the utterance as well as his hearing peer does. PHI's higher processing skills are not in doubt, and yet he is not allowed to use them because of his linguistic model's extraordinarily heavy reliance on his visual skills and modality.

Perhaps, at this stage, two contrasting examples of actual interchanges that took place in the presence of this writer will help elaborate the point in question. In both instances, the task for the children was the same, and each child had suffered a profound hearing loss, but in one case the mother had not as yet received much instruction and in the other case the mother was highly informed.

In the latter instance the child was shown a series of pictures and was asked to find something with which she could cut. She failed. The informed mother then elaborated on a task that the child had been doing the day before. Despite the child's profound hearing loss the mother did not gesture, but reminded the child, through language alone, that she had been cutting and pasting the day before. On seeing that the child remembered, she repeated the question, "What did you cut with?" "Scissors" was the response. The mother then redirected the child's attention to the task at hand and the child immediately pointed to the scissors. The whole interaction was accomplished with language. There was no frustration, merely a quest for understanding, and the success brought a great deal of mutual reinforcement and pleasure.

The other interchange showed a marked contrast. Again, the profoundly deaf child was asked to point—this time to a bird. He failed. The mother then flapped her arms and raised her eyebrows in question. The child successfully pointed to the bird, but there had been no language processing whatsoever and no linking of the spoken word with the extraverbal cues. Compare the amounts of language that the two children—incidentally of the same age—had processed. The latter child is expressively nearly nonverbal. This example should surely demonstrate that, if language competence is to be achieved, language processing must be used.

In treatment of the phonetic element of a child's language a similar malpractice may occur. To most parents the clarity of their child's speech is all important, and PHI's parents are no exception. Even if PHI says a word that is spontaneous and situationally correct, it may be that all the motivational reinforcement (see Chapter 4) with which this experiment has provided him will be spoiled, because, rather than responding to his utterance in the proper manner, the mother stops to correct the phonetic imperfections. As we know from our earlier references to Dale (1976) et al., this may have truly disastrous linguistic implications. With this in mind, there can be no better practice than that outlined by Ling (1976). The articulatory program, which requires the learning of particular subskills for a target coarticulated sound, cannot, at this stage of research, be bettered. It is, however, vital that the parent be informed, for the danger of the child's being taught sounds in isolation is still far too prevalent in the home, in the school, and in the clinic. A regime similar to that outlined in Chapter 4 will, however, lead to articulatory competence without confusing it with the semantic and syntactic components of language. In the case of the partially hearing child, it is vitally important to attend to the hierarchy of subskills that Ling (1976) outlined so explicitly in his text.

READING AND WRITING AS COMPENSATORY TECHNIQUES FOR THE HEARING IMPAIRED

No chapter on the hearing impaired would be complete if the writer did not enter into the ever present controversy about the efficacy of teaching the profoundly deaf early reading and writing skills. In this country, and it is believed most others, there are still few establishments for the hearing impaired that do not depend heavily on the written word. Sadly, this is the case even at kindergarten level. Changing rooms have written names and instructions; there are written labels for colors, numbers, names, and nouns in general. Blackboards are covered with basic written grammar. The same syntactic structures are often written again and again, and yet we know from allied fields that children cannot learn to read until they have internalized their language. Even the popular press has accepted that many illiterate school leavers are handicapped because of deficits in language skills. Once again, it would appear that we set out to handicap the hearing impaired by sticking to methods that have failed even with the hearing child. Once again, it appears that his main problem is what we do to him rather than his handicap. Let us remember Northern and Downs' (1974) accusation that, as hearing educators, we are reluctant to accept the changes that modern research indicates. If we continue to use reading and writing with the prelinguistic child, we are guilty of an offense that is hard to remediate at a later stage. The work of Chovan and McGettan (1971) also suggests that memory and perceptual processes may be hampered if the spoken word is related to the written.

As Ling (1976) has said, few hearing-impaired children read for pleasure. This writer has also observed that few who are taught at too early an age read with comprehension, and none have acquired speech and language skills as a result of their mechanical reading ability. Why is this? Maybe the answer comes from research into the learning-disordered child. Elisabeth Wiig (1976) has shown that adolescents in this group display cognitive, semantic, and linguistic processing deficits. She also discussed the relative importance of short-term/long-term memory skills in overcoming such deficits. In the prelinguistic, partially hearing child, no time has been allowed to acquire semantic and syntactic skills. Furthermore, we have already suggested that short-term memory may be thoroughly overloaded, at least visually, if a simplified form of total communication is being used. If reading is added, this overload can only be exaggerated. Wiig (1976) suggested that, in the processing of syntactic rules, short-term memory skills are of paramount importance. It would seem that the hearing-impaired child is given little chance to learn in the manner for which his innate capacity has programmed him.

Reading and writing are not the answer to the hearing-impaired child's problem, and their early acquisition as "skills" seems to have no recommendations whatsoever. It is difficult to know why their teaching persists. If it is hoped that generalization from reading to language will help in the acquisition of the latter, it has been proved that this is an impossibility. Similarly, if it is believed that because some children are not going to talk they need to read, we know that early reading does not lead to reading for pleasure or to the acquisition of higher reading skills. It is devastating that such outmoded and ill-founded practices can still be witnessed worldwide. Again, it would seem that our hearing-impaired child is less handicapped by his loss than by the chain of events that his loss induces in the behaviors and practices of others. It is hardly surprising that parents resort to the written word in desperation when they believe that their child has not heard or understood. When the "informed" educator is busy teaching with such methods, of course the parent will follow, and yet whoever heard of a normal mother-child linguistic interchange involving the written word with the preschool child? Perhaps it is time for dogmatism: in the light of current research findings, it would seem to be nothing short of criminal to attempt to teach the hearing-impaired child to read and write before or while he is acquiring basic language. However deaf he is, an attempt should be made to develop cognition and language in a manner as nearly approaching the norm as possible.

CONCLUSION

An argument has been presented for the use of audition as the prime modality for language reception, at least initially, and definitely during the critical language learning period, however impaired a child's hearing. The rationale for this has been drawn from allied research fields and from an examination of normal language-learning procedures.

This argument has been generalized to cover the basic theories of the entire text, for it is suggested that the modification of the mother-child interchange is particularly necessary when one is concerned with a child with a hearing loss.

SUMMARY

We discuss in this chapter six areas that must be accepted by every educator of the hearing impaired as possible anxiety producers. These are all variables that may be tackled in therapy with supervised mother-child interactions that are as close to normal as possible. Particular stress is given to the need for PHI to be given the same opportunities to process linguistic information as are given his hearing counterpart, NORM. To do this, PHI must have access to complete linguistic input.

CASE HISTORIES

J. C. (Now Age 19)

This boy (Table 7.1) was referred to the writer at six months of age upon diagnosis of a profound hearing loss. The parents, both

Table 7.1.   Audiometric data (J.C.)

Frequency	125	250	500	1000	2000	4000	8000
Right		110	105	100	110	110	NR*
Left		100	95	100	90	90	NR
Unaided sound field							
Aided sound field		80	80	75	80	80	

* NR = No response at intensity limits of audiometry.

teachers, had not completed adoption formalities but continued with them, although profound deafness had been experienced in their own family. The previous deafness had been managed in the traditional manner through residential school and visually dominant teaching strategies. The child was fitted with two body-worn hearing aids and the parents immediately started guidance as outlined in this text. Although no formal programs were followed, normal language practices were used throughout, and were matched to cognitive data. It was assumed that residual hearing should be the favored modality at all times. Vision was left for the perusal of semantic relationships revealed by situational cues, at least during the first two years of management. Both parents became the agents of habilitation and the prime instigators of all procedures throughout the child's management. Initially, anxiety was a critical factor because of family pressures to follow the traditional education procedures. The parents did not accept that deaf/mutism (as seen before in their relative) was all that the child had potential for and they pursued their own course. They were gradually reinforced by their son's responses and his excellent use of residual hearing. Cognitive and semantic development advanced normally. By four years of age, the child was using short noun phrases and verb phrases in the correct semantic situation. Voicing was good; all vowels and many "low" consonants were present. The child entered normal kindergarten. By seven years this boy could hold a thoroughly normal conversation, although some transformations were still not present at an expressive level. The phoneme /s/ and all its blends were the only severely distorted or substituted sounds; some other blends were spasmodically incorrect. Prosodically, speech was excellent, although there was, and still is, some very slight hypernasality, which might pass as "normal" to the uninformed.

Reading was not delayed, which suggests near normal language skills. The child has been enrolled in normal schools all along, and academic achievement has been above average throughout, allowing for tertiary education. Socially, he has always had friends, but in later years close friendships have not developed and this has caused some distress. Despite apparently negligible hearing, this adult is still heavily dependent on his postauricular aids. He is, however, now a skilled lipreader, but this skill was self-taught and was never introduced as a compensatory technique during the language critical years.

M. G. (Nine Years Old at Time of This Writing)

This child (Table 7.2) was referred at 3½ years of age with grossly aggressive behavior, critically anxious parents, and, as yet, no hearing aids because of a phenomenally late diagnosis. The child was desperately trying to follow advanced visual cues. There had been a constant history of middle ear pathologies (later it was established that this always dramatically reduces hearing). At the time of diagnosis, little language was used between parent and child, and play was impossible. Negative practices by the parents were rife, and the child had become deeply frustrated, hyperactive, and almost impossible to handle. The mother was tearful and admitted to "hating" the child; she was desperate and had a new baby. Stress was evident between the parents because of the child. The child never smiled and was pale and grizzled.

Little M. G. at about this time was fitted with two body aids, and parent guidance was started. The parents were shown how to talk to her by matching the linguistic data with the play situation. They were soon rewarded by a modification in the child's behavior. Hyperactivity was replaced by concentration; tears were replaced by many more smiles. The mother's efforts at a warm, loving, and encouraging approach were rewarded.

At this time it was suggested to the parents by the State authorities that the child enter a kindergarten for the hearing

Table 7.2. Audiometric data (M.G.)

Frequency	125	250	500	1000	2000	4000	8000
Right	20	20	25	50	90	80	75
Left	25	25	35	65	95	NR	NR
Unaided sound field							
Aided sound field							

impaired from 9.00 a.m. to 3.00 p.m. daily. The mother, confident in the newly found relationship, was reluctant to do this, but was critically anxious about what was right. All emphasis, since diagnosis, had been put on audition as the prime modality for language input, with the parents as the language models, and the child was apparently loving this. Kindergarten would mean a visually dominant program with no parental involvement and play companions who had no language. The parents decided on placement in a normal kindergarten at four years. The child, whose behavior was dramatically improved, did not undergo any integration problems and settled immediately and happily. At this time, comprehension through audition was at approximately a three-year-old level and expressive speech was a mass of prosodically meaningful, but articulatorily jumbled, sounds. Voice was completely normal and attempts at expressive speech almost nonstop. At five years of age the child was placed in a normal school where the children accepted her and appeared to understand her, but the teachers still could not understand her grossly deviant speech. By this time it was apparent to the clinician and parents, who nearly always understood her verbalizations, that a good basic linguistic grammar had developed. Also at this time, the mother began to use the language program in a formal manner, and at six years the child was fitted with an F.M. hearing aid, which teachers and parents found invaluable.

At nine years of age the child is coping magnificently, has advanced language, does not rely on lipreading at all, and uses her aided hearing exactly as the normal child uses his hearing.

Speech is good and blends are being gradually generalized from drill techniques into spontaneous speech. Few people realize that this child has anything wrong if she wears her post-auricular aids, with which she can now manage. The F.M. aid is still used in the classroom situation and for speech teaching.

Academically, she is ahead of many of her peers, has no social or behavioral problems, and has a warm relationship with both parents. Occasionally, a negative behavior patch occurs, and this is nearly always associated with the onset of middle ear problems.

G.G.

The history, age, and audiogram of this child is almost exactly the same as the previous one, although hearing over the lower frequencies is slightly less. Behavior, however, was not nearly as severe a problem. Parental anxiety was at a damaging level, and marked compensatory tactics had been used to try to communicate with the completely nonverbal child. The girl was shy, very dependent on mother, and reluctant to try anything that might result in failure.

Following another critically late diagnosis, two body-worn hearing aids were fitted, and progress has been made almost exactly as with the first child. Interestingly, the quantity of language, as measured by M.L.U. (mean length of utterance), was much more restricted in this case at the age of five, although the language was grammatically correct, clear, and easy to follow apart from t/k errors and /s/ blend omissions. Anxiety in the mother at each new academic goal has been a constant problem, but she does recognize it herself. As the child began to read, she anticipated problems, and reading became a dangerous situation at home, as did writing and spelling, until negative reinforcement practices were eradicated. Once the anxiety has been acknowledged, it has always been modifiable through some form of technique demonstrated by the clinician that was positively rewarding to both mother and child.

Note: The parents of both the above girls know each other and occasionally the children have seen each other. There has been much mutual reinforcement and encouragement. The resulting success has been rewarding to all. Each family has acknowledged that they are beginning to think that their problems are in the past, and that now their children's futures will only present them with the more general queries faced by all parents. The children are thought of as hearing children.

A.W. (Now Age Four)

This child (Table 7.3) was referred at the age of 3½ having just been diagnosed as severely hearing impaired. He had already been placed in the full-time kindergarten for hearing-impaired children, where none of his peers were able to speak and where visual compensation was heavily relied upon, although some audition was used. The mother's anxiety had reached pathologic levels and was not only

Table 7.3. Audiometric data (A.W.)

Frequency	125	250	500	1000	2000	4000	8000
Right		60	75	85	85	80	80
Left		60	75	85	85	80	NR
Unaided sound field							
Aided sound field	10	15	35	50	50	50	80

associated with the child's hearing, but also with numerous other family problems. The father had critically high expectations and found it difficult to accept that language was the base for all learning. Preacademic skills appeared to him to be more important than prelinguistic skills. The mother was not receiving counseling from the kindergarten, but there was undoubted relief from the pressure of having to cope with daily behavioral battles, because the child was away from her.

This child had a highly advanced and elaborate gesture system, made no spontaneous vocalizations despite a comparatively mild loss, and riveted much of his attention on the speaker's mouth, regardless of the presence of new and stimulating play material. Despite this habit—which had been taught—it was evident through testing that, when aided, the child had no difficulty in comprehending simple syntactic language through audition alone. After six months, reception was at a normal level, but expression was still minimal. Psychiatric opinion suggested that the compounding problems were so great that the mother would not be a suitable agent for habilitation, nor could normal school placement be entertained.

As a result, continued therapy of a type that was in conflict with his schooling was discontinued. The child remains heavily dependent on gesture and nonverbal cues, as used in communication with his peers. Expressive language constitutes single nouns spoken in a flat voice. The question is, what added traumas will be brought to this child who, when aided, has hearing within normal limits for language acquisition, but who is condemnded to an environment of nonverbal peers? In this writer's opinion, normal kindergarten placement and no therapy at all would have proved a healthier situation; for it is well understood that children conform to the behavior of their peers, and in this case the peers are nonverbal.

M.T. (Age Five)

This child (Table 7.4) has always been described as totally deaf by her mother and has consistently shown complete lack of response through audition. Despite this, and despite some early signs, the mother has always spoken to the child appropriately for her age and cognitive development. Grammatical speech has always been used.

At four, the child was referred to this clinician, and was, at the same time, attending a kindergarten for the hearing impaired in a total communication class.

Although the mother spoke to the child almost normally and comprehension through lipreading was excellent, it was soon

Table 7.4. Audiometric data (M.T.)

Frequency	125	250	500	1000	2000	4000	8000
Right	NR	NR	NR	NR	NR	NR	NR
Left	65	90	NR	NR	NR	NR	NR
Unaided sound field							
Aided sound field							

apparent that the mother did not expect or try to elicit more than a one-word, concrete (noun) answer from her child. The mother was instructed in the use of the language program, and all sections have been worked on. Extended noun phrases and verb phrases are now in the child's expressive grammar, and are correctly ordered. A few transformations are evident. Wh-questions, for example, are understood and used correctly.

M.T.'s speech is limited, but with the use of drills and a heavy dependence on kinesthetic modality, voicing, and voiceless and nasal qualities have been mastered, and many distinctive features are at least evident in the drill. Prosodic stress patterns and duration techniques are also manageable.

It is agreed by all who see this child that her language is far in advance of her peers in her class. It is suggested herein that the reason for this is that her mother has always matched her language to the situational cues and cognitive data and has consistently expanded on language and never limited it.

M.W. (Age 4¾)

This child (Table 7.5) was referred after diagnosis at the age of 2½ years. As is evident from the profound hearing loss, she is extremely handicapped. Initially, she was fitted with two body-worn hearing

Table 7.5. Audiometric data (M.W.)

Frequency	125	250	500	1000	2000	4000	8000
Right		75	80	100	110	NR	NR
Left		75	80	95	100	100	NR
Unaided sound field							
Aided sound field							

aids, but she was soon transferred to an F.M. unit, which assisted the mother as she developed her talking skills. (It is important to realize that such a unit allows a mother to communicate with her child from any distance, while standard aids require proximity for maximum benefit. This feature is of enormous benefit to mothers with young children (Figure 7.6).) M.W. has been severely handicapped by constant middle ear infections, but emphasis has always been on audition. The child makes excellent use of residual hearing, and always indicates if her aids are not working. She does, however, lip-read, but this is a skill that has been self-taught and is only used when the child feels it necessary.

At the time of this writing, the child is showing good comprehension and is "chattering" a great deal with recognizable prosodic patterns. Mother has undergone constant guidance and has an excellent understanding of child development and language. Despite two younger siblings, her anxiety is normal, and a warm and communicative relationship exists. This girl has had a year in a normal kindergarten where the teachers made no special allowances, and where she integrated well and has made a number of neighborhood friendships. The child vocalizes constantly with other children and chatters continuously, but the language is still not comprehensible to others. It is, however, apparent that the child knows exactly what she is saying, and because of the close "link" with the situational circumstances, the listener can compensate and understand. The situation gives the words the child is saying their meaning. It would appear to be a language-learning situation for the listener.

B.M. (Age 11)

This boy (Table 7.6) was referred at four years of age, having received his early education in a kindergarten and then a primary school for the hearing impaired. He could comprehend nothing through aided residual hearing alone, had an advanced gestural com-

Table 7.6. Audiometric data (B.M.)

Frequency	125	250	500	1000	2000	4000	8000
Right	65	75	90	100	100	95	NR
Left	70	75	90	100	105	NR	NR
Unaided sound field							
Aided sound field							

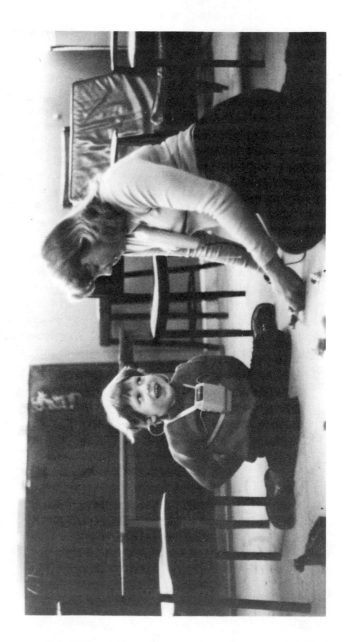

Figure 7.6.   Mother and child using an F.M. hearing aid.

104

municative system, lip-read a great deal, and was an excellent mechanical reader, but showed no comprehension of what he was reading. Expressively, his speech was limited to nouns. Even if asked with lipreading what a person was doing (the questioner pointing to a boy on a bike) the answer would be first "boy" or "bike," but never "riding." His language was entirely concrete and centered on nouns. Upon observation, it was noted that the parents were relying on gesture heavily and using little normal language. Intensive parental guidance and a program based on audition alone have transformed this child into one who can understand advanced syntactic structures through audition alone and who is well intergrated in a normal school. Unfortunately, language development came so late that reading with comprehension is still delayed, and speech skills are limited, but developing fast.

W.S. (Age Four)

This child's hearing loss (Table 7.7) was diagnosed at 15 months of age and appropriate aids were immediately fitted. The parents have always spoken normally to the child, and they received early counseling. At three years she was placed in a play group with hearing children, but with teachers of the deaf to help with her specific problem. Also at three years the parents started learning the language program in this text, the child was fitted with an F.M. hearing aid, and all emphasis was placed on the auditory modality. A sound-teaching drill was started. Both parents have attended sessions regularly, and all "therapy" has been performed through them as agents and language models. At four years, W. has integrated all language structures described in the program, and her spontaneous grammar and speech is excellent, although not all sounds achieved in drills have, as yet, generalized into spontaneous speech. This child is now at the stage when few realize that she has a problem (when she is wearing concealed postauricular aids). She will enter normal school at the normal age.

Table 7.7. Audiometric data (W.S.)

Frequency	125	250	500	1000	2000	4000	8000
Right	NR	70	80	90	110	95	NR
Left	NR	100	110	NR	NR	NR	NR
Unaided sound field							
Aided sound field							

REFERENCES

Brown, R. 1977. The place of baby talk in the world of language. In: C. Snow and C. Ferguson (eds.), Talking to Children. Cambridge University Press, New York.

Chovan, W. I., and J. F. McGettan. 1971. The effects of vocal mediating responses on visual motor tasks with deaf and hearing children. Except. Child 37:435–438.

Cornett, R. O. 1967. Cued speech. Am. Ann. Deaf 112:3–13.

Dale, P. S. 1976. Language Development: Structure and Function, 2nd Ed. Holt, Rinehart & Winston, New York.

Goldstein, M. A. 1939. The Acoustic Method for the Training of the Deaf and Hard of Hearing child. Laryngoscopic Press, St. Louis.

Ivimey, G. O. 1976. The written syntax of an English deaf child: An exploration in method. BJDC 11(2):103–120.

Kimura, D. 1963. Right temporal lobe damage, perception of unfamiliar stimuli after damage. Arch. Neurol. 8:264–271.

Ling, D. 1976. Speech and the Hearing-Impaired Child: Theory and Practice. Alexander Graham Bell Association for the Deaf, Washington, D.C.

Luria, A. R. 1976. The Working Brain. Penguin Books, New York.

Newport, E. L., H. Gleitman, and L. R. Gleitman. 1977. I'd rather do it myself. Some effects and non effects of maternal speech styles. In: C. Snow and C. Ferguson (eds.), Talking to Children. Cambridge University Press, New York.

Northern, J. L., and M. P. Downs. 1974. Hearing in Children. Williams & Wilkins Co., Baltimore.

Owrid, H. L. 1977. Auditory and visual communication, the work of Bernard Trevoort. BJDC 12(1):61–67.

Pollack, E., and N. Rees. 1972. Disorders of articulation. Some clinical implications of distinctive feature theory. JSHD 37(4):451–461.

Silverman, S. R., and H. Davis. 1970. Hard of Hearing Children. Hearing and Deafness, 3rd Ed. Holt, Rinehart & Winston, New York.

Sussman, H. 1972. What the tongue tells the brain. Psychol. Bull. 77(4):262–272.

Wedenberg, E. 1951. Auditory training of deaf and hard of hearing children. Acta Otolaryngol. (suppl.) 94.

Whetnall, E., and D. B. Fry. 1971. The Deaf Child. Charles C Thomas, Springfield, Illinois.

Wiig, E. 1976. Language disabilities of adolescents. BJDC 11(1):3–17.

Chapter 8

Application to Hearing Assessment, Hearing-Aid Evaluation and Hearing-Aid Orientation

Ronald J. Balthazor

Children spend more time with their parents than with any other being during the first few years of their lives. Besides their enormous time commitment, parents are the most familiar with the child's likes and dislikes in toys, food, clothes, and people. In addition, parents are probably the most motivated, most enthusiastic, and the most viable agents in the training of their children. To assist with the management of a partially hearing child, practical suggestions are made that will enable the parents to maximize the use of the child's auditory channel in the acqustion of speech and language. The application of these suggestions is limited to the young, partially hearing, preverbal child (infant to four-year-old). The basis on which the suggestions are made is fourfold. First, the child has an innate capacity to learn language (Lenneberg, 1967) and no hearing impairment can preclude that capacity. Second, every partially hearing child has some degree of useable hearing (Elliott, 1967; Hine, 1973; Montgomery, 1967). Third, hearing is the only temporally based sensory system ideally suited to perceiving speech (Liberman et al., 1967). Fourth, the parents play a crucial role in taking advantage of that useable hearing during the years vital to language development (Halle, 1964; Tervoort, 1964).

IDENTIFICATION

In a previous chapter, reference is made to the anxious mother. Her anxiety exists because of a breakdown in the chain of communication, and nowhere is it more evident than during the initial visit to the speech and hearing center, when the parents have begun to suspect a hearing deficiency in their child. They are aware that "deafness" has profound effects on the child's ability to talk, and that their child does not seem to respond to sound. Most importantly, they are aware that their child does not behave "normally."

Many parents live with these suspicions for long periods of time (Malkin et al., 1976). Some parents are ultimately referred for a speech and hearing evaluation of their child by other professionals, and some parents come to the center either out of sheer desperation caused by professional rejection of their suspicions or out of frustration with the recommendation that "He'll grow out of it." Irrespective of the reason for the first clinical visit, suspicions and anxiety exist. To reduce these hurdles to parental involvement and cooperation, it is essential that anxiety be diagnosed as either normal or pathological and be dealt with appropriately. This diagnosis is the first step toward confident and respectful interaction between parents and professionals. The clinician's ability to differentiate between the various anxiety levels will allow her to deal suitably with the parent should the assessment of hearing finally confirm the parental suspicion of a hearing loss. This ability will also reduce the probability of time-consuming and emotionally draining searches for second, third, and fourth opinions.

Initial attempts at the alleviation of anxiety are best begun during the case-history interview. Here, the most essential information may not be the identification of possible contributing factors to the child's hearing impairment but rather the identification of underlying reasons for the parental suspicion and anxiety. Case-history data are not simply critical milestones used for contrast with normative data but, more importantly, are observations for which the parents should receive positive feedback. Their ability to report various behaviors, such as reaction to sounds, social interactions, and quantitative and qualitative vocalization, will be useful for the ongoing assessment of hearing, hearing aid selection, and therapeutic progress.

Audiologic evaluation should be consistent with the case-history information. With the extremely young, however, this may be difficult to achieve. Audiologic correlation may only be made with the risk factors stated in a high-risk register (National Joint Committee, 1973). For the older infant, points of consistency may be easier to determine. This consistency should be indicated to the parents, not only because it relates to establishing the site and the effects of hearing loss, but also because it locates the source of parental suspicion and possible anxiety. More constructively, it establishes with some reliability the ability of the parents to monitor behavior critical to the future development of their child.

In addition to the role they play in the case-history stage of the identification process, parents may also have an integral involvement in the actual audiologic assessment. This role may be passive of necessity if electrophysiologic diagnostic procedures are employed. The parent's role can be a more active one if Conditioned Orientation Reflex (Suzuki and Ogiba, 1961), Tangible Reinforcement Operant Conditioning (Lloyd, 1968, Bricker and Bricker, 1969), Peep Show (Dix and Halpike, 1947), Pup Show (Green, 1958), Visual Reinforcement (Liden and Kankkonen, 1961), or Play Audiometry (Lloyd, 1966) procedures are used. The value of either passive or active participation by the parents is based, of course, on their understanding of the test and its rationale. Understanding is critical if the parent is to serve, for example, as a reinforcing agent in Play Audiometry. Often parents are required to provide a nonresponsive lap in Conditioned Orientation Reflex (COR) or Tangible Reinforcement Operant Conditioning Audiometry (TROCA). In COR, TROCA, or Play Audiometry a basis for eventual therapeutic models and behavior modification is being laid. The audiometric stimulus-response-consequation (S-R-C) paradigm should therefore be utilized to create an understanding of the potential this technique has for shaping the desired behavior of the child.

If parents have an understanding of test purposes, test rationale, and test techniques, the diagnostic results are more readily acceptable to them. Understanding of the S-R-C paradigm can also aid in an explanation of the breakdown in the communication chain. Consideration and feeling should be used when explaining the results of the audiologic evaluation to the parents. With the child for whom assessment confirms the suspicion of hearing impairment, the results may not be exactly what the parents wanted to hear. These instances are more tactfully handled by confirming the observations of the parents rather than by simply interpreting the audiologic data. Since additional visits may be necessary to refine the initial assessment, and only parental cooperation will ensure an ultimately valid diagnosis, great care must be taken to win the parents' confidence.

MEDICAL MANAGEMENT

Following the audiologic determination of a hearing loss, the child should be referred for a medical evaluation. This is necessary for three reasons. The first is to determine any potential medical or surgical remediation of the hearing loss. The second is to provide medically oriented counseling regarding the role of the physician in relation to the particular type of hearing loss. The third is to eliminate any contraindications to amplification or earmold usage should the pathology not be amenable to medical treatment. Communication among the medical profession, the parent, and the clinician are crucial for the hearing-impaired child. Besides providing the confirmation of the hearing loss, the medical practitioner may be frequently called upon to provide additional services. In an investigation of deaf children, Malkin et al. (1976) found that such youngsters have a higher rate of tonsillectomy and adenoidectomy procedures (40.9%) than is normal for the general population of similar age (0.17%–2.0%). In addition, these authors found that 14.5% of deaf patients also required myringotomies. Such findings suggest that medical contact may be more frequent than that required for a normal-hearing child, and both the medical practitioner and parent should be aware of the implications that associated pathologies may have on the child's auditory sensitivity. Even a slight conductive component produced by an upper respiratory tract infection and overlaid on a severe sensorineural hearing loss may preclude the only benefits provided by amplification. Closer medical and audiologic care in the child's total management is therefore demanded as part of an appropriate surveillance program.

EFFECTS OF HEARING LOSS

Audiometric results are the best initial step in any explanation of the effects of hearing loss. The frequency × intensity plot of the audiogram provides an indication of the child's reduced hearing sensitivity. Most important is the realization that sensitivity is reduced for some frequencies more than for others. This change in the normal intensity relationships between low, medium, and high frequencies creates a degree of distortion in the perception of the signal. Two other common sensory aberrations associated with a sensorineural hearing loss are added to the interactive distortion produced by frequency-dependent sensitivity reductions. First, a reduction in the ear's ability to tolerate loud sounds may also be associated with reduced sensitivity. This parallel reduction in sensitivity and tolerance may restrict the dynamic range or the range of useful hearing to 10–30 dB (Erber, 1973). Second, the sensorineural ear may require a greater period of time to collect the necessary neural information required for auditory processing. This reduction in temporal summation or integration has been explored by several investigators (Barry and Larson, 1974; Gengel and Watson, 1971; Sanders and Honig, 1967; Singh and Greenberg, 1976; Wright, 1968) and can be used as a differentiating factor in the diagnosis of a sensorineural hearing loss. The effects of frequency, intensity, and temporal distortions on the child's speech perception are not straightforward. Speech discrimination depends on the perception of all three variables, but their complex interaction makes determination of the essential speech cues difficult. Predicting speech discrimination abilities from audiometric data is problematic (Elliott, 1963). However, a basic understanding of speech acoustics will develop an appreciation of speech as a complex, multidimensional act dependent upon some degree of hearing for perception.

Speech is essentially an acoustic representation resulting from the effects that vocal tract configuration has on the signal source generated with or without laryngeal vibrations. The individual speech sounds, vowels, and consonants are composed of concentrations of acoustic energy within select frequency ranges. Figure 8.1 depicts a frequency × intensity × time recording (called a speech spectrogram) of the utterance, "She should make Sam a sandwich." Frequency is displayed along the ordinate. Intensity is shown by the various degrees of shading—the darker the shading, the greater the intensity. Time is linearly represented along the axis. The distinct bands reflect the energy concentrations, or formants, that compose the individual speech sounds. In the typical sensorineural hearing loss the sensitivity for the higher frequencies is reduced markedly from the sensitivity for the lower frequencies. To depict this effect, the upper-half, higher frequency components of the speech spectrogram can be covered. This shows the reduction of frequency information in the speech signal but does not show reduction or alteration in the intensity for the lower frequencies and the effects of any temporal distortion within the ear.

To ensure that the partially hearing child is provided with the maximal use of his auditory system, it is necessary to reduce, as much as possible, the distortions that the hearing disorder imposes. For those with a sensorineural hearing loss, amplification is the only means that will reduce the distortion in the speech signal produced by unequal frequency emphasis. Only through the use of amplification, initiated at as early an age as possible, can advantage be taken of the critical language-learning period (Tervoort, 1964). Maximal use of residual hearing during this period will improve the probability that the child will not develop significant secondary social, educational, vocational, and psychologic problems.

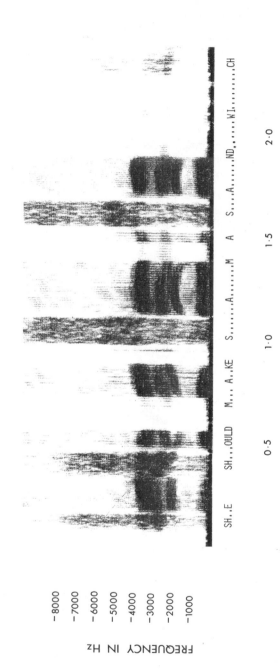

Figure 8.1. A speech spectrogram of the sentence "She should make Sam a sandwich."

IMPORTANCE OF AMPLIFICATION

For the child with a sensorineural hearing loss severe enough to interfere with the normal acquisition of speech and language, few corrective measures are available. The personal hearing aid is the most predominantly selected means of remediation. In essence, any hearing aid is composed of three basic components, which are illustrated in Figure 8.2. The microphone collects airborne or acoustic energy and converts it into electrical energy. The amplifier receives the weak electrical impulses from the microphone and increases the signal strength. Boosted electrical energy from the amplifier is then converted back into acoustic energy by the earphone (receiver in hearing aid terminology) for channeling into the ear canal via a custom-made earmold. This electronic system, like a public address system, simply makes sounds louder. All sounds, not just speech, are amplified by such a device.

The importance of this amplification lies in what making sounds louder can do to bring the range of speech (40-80 dB SPL) within the child's hearing sensitivity and to lessen, to a degree, the distortion produced by frequency-dependent loudness reductions. The earlier this use of the child's residual hearing capability is initiated, the more benefits he can derive. Elliott and Armbruster (1967) suggest that additional learning handicaps may result from a delay in early amplification and training. This potential risk in delaying habilitative measures is highlighted by a study in which visual deprivation in kittens resulted in alterations in the physiologic function of their sensory system after only three to six weeks (Wiesel and Hubel, 1965).

It is necessary to explain to the parents, however, that amplification cannot restore hearing to a normal or even near normal state. No hearing aid can perfectly compensate for the pattern of a sensory deficit, because the hearing aid has its own intrinsic distortions and limitations (Schweitzer, Causey, and Tolton, 1977; Bode and

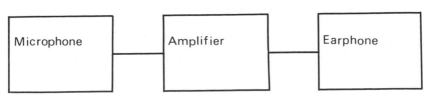

Figure 8.2.   A block diagram of the three major hearing aid components: microphone, amplifier, and earphone.

Kasten, 1971; Kasten and Lotterman, 1967). These limitations are imposed by the design of electronic components as well as by the hearing loss itself.

Restrictions in the dynamic range of the sensorineural ear, produced by concurrent reductions in sensitivity and levels of tolerance, may create a very narrow range of usable hearing. The ability of a hearing aid to make sounds louder (gain) and, yet, not too loud (maximum power output) must fall within the reduced dynamic range. The hearing aid must also provide this amplification across the widest possible range of frequencies (bandwidth) affected by the hearing loss.

The degree to which matching electroacoustic characteristics of the hearing aid to the hearing loss can be successfully achieved determines the amount of favorable habilitative prognosis. Even in cases of severe or profound hearing loss, benefits from aural remediation can occur with the present amplification potential, the redundancies in language, and the varieties of aural habilitation programs.

Redundancy of speech and language occurs at many levels. Language, for instance, is composed of phonologic, morphologic, syntactic, and semantic components. These components are arranged in ordered strings to express thoughts, intentions, experiences, or feelings. The rules that govern their order place definite limitaions on the potential variability of an utterance after it is begun. Once learned, these linguistic rules enable the listener to decode entire utterances based on incomplete information. How much the learning of these rules is ultimately dependent upon hearing is not fully known, and although the redundancy of language makes its perception a robust phenomenon, some perception of the speech signal must be present to facilitate the rule acquisition.

Various studies (Hirsh, Reynolds, and Joseph, 1954; French and Steinburg, 1947;) have indicated that good speech intelligibility can be achieved with only certain portions of the speech spectrum. Eighty-eight percent of all children enrolled at the Central Institute for the Deaf were reported to respond to the pure-tone testing frequency of 2000 Hz within the limits of the audiometric equipment (Elliott, 1967). All children could respond to the 1000 Hz test tone. If, for instance, an analysis is made of the spectral information in speech at or below 2000 Hz, which is available to a majority of the partially hearing children, it can be determined how many acoustic cues do exist.

The first and second formants of most vowels fall below 2000 Hz. Added to these cues for vowel identification (Peterson and Barney,

1952), the second formant transitions produced by adjacent consonants will also be present. These transitions have been identified as information carried by the vowel that is sufficient for identification of the adjacent consonants (Liberman et al., 1967; Martin, Pickett, and Colten, 1972). In addition, cues associated with vowel perception also reveal phonemic, dialectical, and other paralinguist information (Fairbanks and Grubb, 1961; Ladefoged and Broadbent, 1957).

The temporal patterning of the lower pitched components, including the fundamental frequency, when perceived in conjunction with the varying durations and stresses of successive syllables, provides prosodic information, which can help, for instance, in differentiating between sentences that make a statement, ask a question, or require syntactic disambiguating (Lehiste, Olive, and Streeter, 1976).

The above factors should highlight the importance of perceiving the frequency components of speech below approximately 2000 Hz. With the degree of information provided through amplification, the partially hearing child should have an excellent prognosis for developing speech and language when audition is complemented by appropriate habilitative training, as suggested by Ling (1976).

HEARING-AID EVALUATION

There are a variety of test procedures and test stimuli employed in the selection of an individual hearing aid. Without going into a discussion of the philosophic bases of evaluation procedures, this section points out considerations in the selection process that will enable the parents to become as independent as possible in the management of their partially hearing child.

As with the various audiometric methods previously discussed, parental participation can play an important role in hearing-aid evaluation. Again, focus is directed on the S-R-C paradigm that is employed in the majority of testing situations. Exposing the parents to this method can highlight the behavior modification techniques that will be an essential tool in the speech and language development of the child. In addition, parental participation, perhaps in the capacity of providing positive reinforcement, allows the parent to experience a variety of testing stimuli. Active parental presence in the sound-field testing situation can provide a dramatic demonstration (for the parent) of the child's hearing abilities. Stimulus intensity levels required for criterion responses can be contrasted in the aided and unaided testing conditions. Not only can these contrasts emphasize the importance of amplification in improving the child's range of hearing sensitivity, but they can also serve as a basis for refining the parent's skills in observing the child's auditory behavior. These observation skills will be critical for the ongoing evaluation process. This progressive evaluation allows for the monitoring and determination of the benefits of amplification for the child and also helps to determine the appropriateness of the initially selected electroacoustic characteristics of the hearing aid.

Following the formal hearing-aid evaluation procedures, it is suggested that more informal procedures be utilized. Even having the child simply identify and discriminate a variety of sounds such as /i/, /e/, /s/, and /ʃ/ would be sufficient for establishing an indication of hearing-aid function. Such procedures can be employed routinely by the parent or by the therapist outside the formal testing situation. More importantly, they establish the benefits of the selected hearing aid and enable those benefits to be monitored throughout the child's day.

During the hearing-aid evaluation, attention should be paid to the accumulation of results. Progressive interpretation to the parents of the findings underscores the importance of and the prognosis for amplification. Gradual provision of information decreases parental confusion when the final hearing aid is selected.

Following the selection of a hearing aid, the parents should be introduced to means that will provide information helpful to the refinement of the initial hearing aid selection, and the beneficial use of the instrument by the child. These goals can be accomplished with the use of formal recording sheets (Alpiner, 1975; Clark, 1975; and Smith, 1975) or by making individual modifications as they are found necessary for each particular circumstance.

HEARING-AID ORIENTATION

Orientation is a process of counseling, demonstration, and practice that has as its main objective the optimal usefulness of the hearing aid. This seems a simple goal, but it requires all the sensitivity and expertise that the professional can muster. The usefulness of the hearing aid depends not only on establishing a working knowledge of components and controls but also on an understanding of the effects of hearing loss, the importance of amplification, and the establishment of parental cooperation based on motivation and mutual respect for the management team.

The basis, therefore, for the orientation program is laid during the initial clinical visit and is built up over time during the hearing assessment and hearing-aid selection procedures. Unlike the hearing-air orientation programs for adults, the reinforcement provided the child by the beneficial aspects of amplification are not experienced by the same person who is responsible for the care and maintenance of the instrument. The active involvement of parents suggested during the hearing and hearing-aid evaluations helps establish for them the importance of the hearing aid for their child. Hopefully motivated by the often dramatic improvement in their child's auditory behavior, parents can be more reliably expected to ensure the maintenance of their child's aid.

The value of establishing full parental cooperation cannot be stressed enough. As managers of the first hearing aid, they will soon encounter many difficulties that would thwart the poorly prepared. This is highlighted by the investigations of Porter (1973), Zink (1972), and Gaeth (1966), all of whom found that approximately 50% of the children enrolled in several schools for the deaf were not receiving the benefits of their hearing aids. Although there were a variety of reasons for such unsuccessful use of amplification in these longitudinal studies, most problems could be attributed to simple malfunctions. These malfunctions would presumably be obvious in even a cursory inspection of batteries, cords, controls, earphones, and earmolds.

No hearing aid can be useful if it is not working, is not working properly, or is not being worn. Maintaining the proper functioning of the instrument can be a challenging task. Parents should expect and hopefully be prepared for the fact that the child's hearing aid and earmold may be stepped on, flushed down, chewed up, thrown across, dropped out, broken apart, hammered with, crushed between, dragged through, dipped in, dribbled upon, sprayed over, and glued together at almost any time. Some of these occurrences may be the usual fate suffered by most objects that the child handles. Other destructive occurrences, however, may be a result of the child's lack of acceptance of the hearing aid. In either case, the parent must be prepared to manage the situation and, where possible, maintain the usefulness of the aid.

The child may not be the only source of challenge to the parent. Frustrations and annoyance can be experienced during the acquisition of the hearing aid. There are usually several avenues available for procuring a hearing aid; government agencies, university or private clinics, commercial dealers, and charitable organizations are all distributors. Each has its own particular referral procedures, financial arrangements, and potential headaches. Those procurement avenues common to each geographic area should be adequately studied by the clinician. Familiarity with local options will prove invaluable when directing parents.

The dispensing agency may or may not provide information regarding the use and maintenance of the hearing aid. Whether parents have been given instructions or not, the clinician should plan on familiarizing the parents with the hearing aid's controls and its maintenance. It is beyond the scope of this chapter to discuss in detail the enormous range of hearing-aid fittings. This topic is treated satisfactorily elsewhere (Pollack, 1975; Hodgson and Skinner, 1977). To some extent, variables related to the choice of hearing-aid fittings determine the number and complexity of the controls, therefore a general discussion of components and associated terminology is in order here.

The *microphone, amplifier,* and *earphone* described earlier in this chapter depend of course, on a power supply for their operation. This is provided by the *battery.* (In rare instances there may even be two batteries.) The size and location of the battery and its compartment depend, in general, on the size of the hearing aid itself, e.g., in body- versus head-worn hearing aids.

The *volume control* is a wheel that can be rotated to alter the amount of amplification provided by the aid. On some hearing aids, rotating the wheel completely in the direction of lower volume will result in a click for the *off position.* The off position on other aids may be incorporated in another control, and in some there may be no off position. In this case the battery contacts must be separated to eliminate battery drainage. Use of the volume control is primarily dependent on the degree of hearing loss and secondarily dependent on the listening situation. A convenience that is not always present is numbering or color shading on the volume control, which enables rapid readjustment to a comfortable listening level.

The *tone control* is used to emphasize certain frequencies of the hearing aid's bandwidth. This is accomplished by altering the frequency response of the amplifier. This control may also incorporate the on/off switch. In most head-worn hearing aids where a tone control is present, it is set by the distributor. Unlike the relatively inaccessible position of the head-worn aid's tone control, the tone control is very prominent on the body-worn hearing aid. The appropriate setting should be checked regularly in case of "accidental" tampering by the child.

Another switch that may also incorporate the on/off control is the *input selector.* The input selector allows for the use of the microphone and/or telephone coil. The telephone coil enables the hearing-aid user to take advantage of stray electromagnetic energy present in the telephone receiver without the interference of ambient room noise. Many hearing aids do not provide this facility, and consequently the input selector would not be present.

The *earmold* provides the coupling between the hearing aid and the ear. In essence, it provides a channel through which acoustic energy is directed into the ear canal. The earmold is an integral part of the hearing-aid system, as it may serve:

1. As an additional means of modifying the acoustic response of the amplified sound
2. As a means of holding body-aid earphones or head-worn aids in place
3. As a critical component in preventing acoustic feedback— hearing aid squeal—in high gain instruments

The earmold may be attached to the hearing aid with plastic *tubing,* as in the case of head-worn instruments. This tubing conveys the acoustic output of the internal earphone to the earmold. In body-worn aids a *cord* carries the electrical output of the hearing aid to an external earphone. The external earphone is then attached to the earmold by means of a snap-ring *connector.*

Transmitters are components associated with the radio-frequency, wearable auditory training units, a specific type of hearing aid. The transmitters serve as a remote wireless microphone that can be used in conjunction with the environmental or internal microphones of the body-worn, radio *receiver.* In this application, cords are also used to carry the electrical signal to external earphones.

Patience is the key word in discussing and demonstrating to the parents the various components and controls of the hearing aid. Sufficient time and appointments should be allowed for repetition of instructions and parental practice, and this should occur relatively early in the parental contact. Thoughts of their child's handicap, its effects, and, now, the visible burden of the hearing aid itself may be overwhelming. It is difficult for parents to concentrate on fine details when the broad complexities of their child's life are before them.

Once the parents have a basic understanding of the hearing aid itself, they will need to know a little about how it runs and how to keep it running. Trouble shooting procedures will be essential if the parents are to manage those episodes of pandemonium produced by hearing-aid malfunction. The procedures can vary from relatively simple listening and visual inspection to more electronically oriented inspection (Eubanks, 1977a, 1977b, 1978). Irrespective of the level of proficiency that the parents might ultimately achieve, the essentials should be learned first. These can then be complemented over time when the parents are more familiar with the aid.

The first concern is with the earmold. Parents should be facile with earmold placement. For this reason, and for the purpose of listening to the aid, it is advisable to have an earmold made for the parent at the same time one is made for the child. Parents can then practice earmold placement on themselves to establish a confident approach when placing it in the child's ear. A properly made earmold, once correctly seated in the ear, should preclude any acoustic feedback. If it does not, the acoustic sealing characteristics can be simply checked by placing a finger over the sound channel while the aid is full on. Feedback under these conditions would indicate that the acoustic leak is coming, not from a poorly seated or ill-fitting earmold, but rather from other hearing-aid/earmold connections or connectors:

1. Tubing to earmold
2. Aid to tubing
3. External earphone to earmold

Hearing aid squeal may be a product of other souces of feedback. The cause of these sources, however, demands correction by the manufacturer.

Earmolds can also be a source of physical irritation. The child may be allergic to the earmold materials themselves or be sensitive to "high" or rough spots in the finished earmold. In either case, reddening and even laceration of the ear will be apparent. These irritations may be alleviated by either buffing or making a new earmold of nonallergenic materials.

Batteries are the next major source of concern. Most aids indicate the way in which the position of the positive terminal of the battery should be located. Each battery should be used until it is exhausted, eliminating the possibility that a half-used battery will become mixed with fresh stock. It is wise to maintain a simple score card of battery life, as it can provide useful information not only on the batteries themselves but also on unusually high drainage by the aid. Increases in battery turnover, then, should raise suspicions about the freshness of the batteries or increases in volume requirements. A small supply of batteries should be maintained, preferably in the refrigerator to reduce aging. It is also a wise practice to remove batteries from the hearing aid when it is not in use. This not only prevents drainage, which occurs even when the aid is off, but also allows for the monitoring of any corrosive build-up. Such build-up can be removed by rubbing with either paper or a pencil eraser. Batteries should not be put in the hearing aid if they appear deformed or are leaking in any way.

Common sense also suggests that battery removal or insertion (or, for that matter, any inspection of the aid) should occur over a stand or table. How disconcerting it must be to reflexively catch a dropped battery or earmold at the expense of a shattered hearing aid!

Once earmold and battery care have been explained, demonstrated, and practiced, parents can listen to the hearing aid. Any scratchiness, intermittency, or feedback, produced by altering the various controls, tubing, or cords should be reported to the clinician. In some instances these can be remedied by replacing tubing or cords, by using contact cleaner on the various controls, or by manipulation of cord prongs and receptacles. These maintenance procedures should be mutually explored by parent and clinician. Attacking problems as they occur will eventually build the independent troubleshooting competence of the parent and will help to ensure useful amplification.

Listening checks can also provide a quick survey of the overall function of the hearing aid. Parents gradually become accustomed to the "sound" of the hearing aid. Any changes in the quality of amplification can subsequently be explored. An interesting method to facilitate these listening checks is provided by Randolph (1976). He suggests coupling the earphone of the hearing aid to the microphone of a cassette recorder. Parents can then easily record speech as it is transduced by the aid. Such recordings provide the potential for comparing the aid's output performance between its initial functioning and that of its routine operation or its operation after repair. It also solves the problem of trying to monitor aid quality while simultaneously speaking and being "traumatized" by the aid's output.

Another recent asset to parental hearing-aid troubleshooting is a unit by Roeser et al. (1977). HAMDU, or hearing-aid malfunction detection unit, is an electronic device that is coupled to a body-worn hearing aid. Every 26 minutes it samples aspects of the electric output of the hearing aid. Any discrepancy in aid function from preset levels triggers an electromagnetic indicator. Such a device, when perfected, will offer significant benefit to maintaining aids in proper working condition.

Troubleshooting of equpiment is, however, only one step in a proper problem solving orientation. Two other major areas of concern are those presented by the number of different communication situations and the acceptance of the aid by the child. Both of these areas must be dealt with to establish the usefulness of the hearing aid.

Communication situations can be affected by the environment, the speaker, and the child himself. Although it is impossible to control all of the parameters associated with these variables, a few considerations should be stressed. The most important aspect of the communication situation is the signal to noise ratio (S/N). This ratio reflects the degree to which the signal (usually speech is the signal critical to the evaluation) is louder than the noise. The signal must be preceptible from within a background of noise for the child to make use of it. Figure 8.3 illustrates the effects of background noise on the spectrographic recording of the sentence, "She should make Sam a sandwich." The difference in the visual clarity of the message can be contrasted with the same sentence uttered without background noise in Figure 8.1. The actual effects on auditory clarity would depend on several factors:

1. The frequency components in the noise
2. The frequency components in the speech
3. Temporal factors of the noise
4. The S/N ratio
5. Several linguistic factors

Several investigators (Gengel, 1971; Olsen and Tillman, 1968; Tillman et al., 1970) have demonstrated that persons with a sensorineural hearing loss require a better S/N ratio than do normal-hearing persons. This emphasizes the importance of assuring the best S/N ratio for the partially hearing child who is trying to learn language, the child who, as yet does not have the linguistic rules that could assist him in extracting meaning from a signal disregarding background noise.

There are a few measures that parents or the clinician can employ to provide the maximal S/N ratio for their child. The most obvious is to reduce the level of background noise, which may require the installation of curtains and rugs for acoustic damping or the removal of the noise generators (sometimes called brothers and sisters) in the primary rooms used for the structured speech and language lessons. Not so obvious a solution is to move the signal source closer to the microphone than the noise. For most hearing aids this requires the speaker to move closer to the child on whom

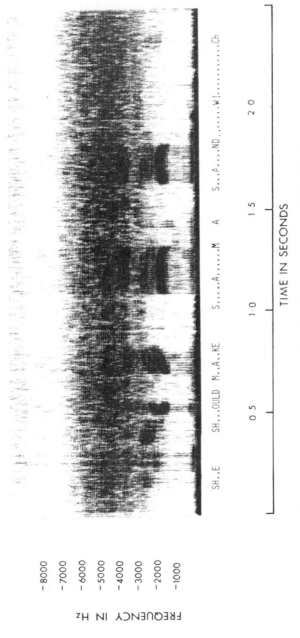

Figure 8.3. A speech spectrogram of the sentence "She should make Sam a sandwich," with a background of noise.

123

the microphone is placed. On radio-frequency hearing aids, the microphone/transmitter is placed on the speaker and has the advantage of always maximizing the S/N ratio.

Modification of the speaker and child variables in the communication situation is the particular concern of this text elsewhere. Little attention will, therefore, be given to them here. However, the critical aspect in the communication situation between mother and child is the hearing aid. Its benefit to communication can only be achieved if it is worn. This will depend on the mutual acceptance of the aid by both mother and child.

Provided that the maximum power output of the hearing aid does not exceed the tolerance levels of the child and that the earmold is not abrasive to the ear, the acceptance of the hearing aid by the child is probably greatly dependent on its acceptance by the parent. Parents who have understood the need for amplification are rarely faced with the quandary posed by having the child make his handicap visible by wearing a hearing aid. They also are well motivated to learn all that is required in the care, maintenance, and placement of the hearing aid. These are the parents who can approach the child in a confident manner and make the constant wearing of the hearing aid no more traumatic than wearing a seat belt. Both the sensory and the safety aid will be accepted by the child if handled in this way.

Acceptance by the parent is a continual influence on the acceptance by the child. The parent who confronts family, friends, or acquaintances with the need and importance of this visible sensory aid will have less trouble with the child rejecting the aid either initially or later during the self-conscious teen years.

SUMMARY

Practical suggestions are provided in this chapter that will assist in establishing the parents as beneficial agents in the audiologic management of the partially hearing child. This active parental role begins with the realization of their abilities to contribute to the aural habilitation program. Such contributions are made by parental observation and by monitoring the child's auditory behavior, and they continue throughout the years of training. Gradually, the parents become the primary managers of the child's hearing aid just as they become the primary agents in the speech and language environment.

REFERENCES

Alpiner, J. 1975. Hearing and selection for adults. In: M. Pollack (ed.), Amplification for the Hearing-Impaired. Grune & Stratton, New York.

Barry, S., and V. Larson. 1974. Brief-tone audiometry with normal and deaf school-age children. J. Sp. Hear. Dis. 39:457-464.

Bode, D., and R. Kasten. 1971. Hearing and distortion and consonant identification. J. Sp. Hear. Res. 14:323-331.

Bricker, D., and W. Bricker. 1969. A programmed approach to operant audiometry for low-functioning children. J. Sp. Hear. Dis. 34:312-320.

Clark, T. (ed.) 1975. Programming for Hearing Impaired Infants Through Amplification. Utah State University, Logan.

Dix, M., and C. Halpike. 1947. The peep show. A new technique for pure-tone audiometry in young chidren. Br. Med. J. 2:712-723.

Elliott, L. 1963. Prediction of speech discrimination scores from other test information. J. Aud. Res. 3:35-45.

Elliott, L. 1967. Descriptive analysis of audiometric and psychometric scores of students at a school for the deaf. J. Sp. Hear. Res. 10:21-40.

Elliott, L., and V. Armbruster. 1967. Some possible effects of the delay of early treatment of deafness. J. Sp. Hear. Res. 10:209-224.

Erber, N. 1973. Body-baffle and real-ear effects in the selection of hearing aids for deaf children. J. Sp. Hear. Dis. 38:224 231.

Eubanks, R. 1977a. A remedy for hearing aid distortion. Audiol. Hear. Ed. 3:15-36.

Eubanks, R. 1977b. Technician tips. Audiol. Hear. Ed. 3:33-36.

Eubanks, R. 1978. Technician tips. Audiol. Hear. Ed. 4:24-26.

Fairbanks, G., and P. Grubb. 1961. A psychophysical investigation of vowel formants. J. Sp. Hear. Res. 4:203-219.

French, N., and J. Steinburg. 1947. Factors governing the intelligibility of speech sounds. J. Acoust. Soc. Am. 19:90-119.

Gaeth, J., and E. Lounsbury. 1966. Hearing aids and children in elementary schools. J. Sp. Hear. Dis. 31:283-289.

Gengel, R. 1971. Acceptable speech-to-noise ratios for aided speech discrimination by the hearing-impaired. J. Aud. Res. 11:219-222.

Gengel, R., and C. Watson. 1971. Temporal integration: I. Clinical implications of a laboratory study. II. Additional data from hearing-impaired subjects. J. Sp. Hear. Dis. 36:213-224.

Green, D. 1958. The pup-show: A simple, inexpensive modification of the peep show. J. Sp. Hear. Dis. 23:118-120.

Halle, M. 1964. The acquisition of language. Child. Dev. Mon. No. 92:29(1).

Haung, O., P. Baccaro, and F. Guilford. 1967. A pure-tone audiogram on the infant: The PIWI technique. Arch. Otolaryngol. 86:101-106.

Hine, W. 1973. How deaf are deaf children? Br. J. Audiol. 7:41-44.

Hirsh, I., E. Reynolds, and M. Joseph. 1954. Intelligibility of different speech materials. J. Acoust. Soc. Am. 26:530-538.

Hodgson, W., and P. Skinner (eds.). 1977. Hearing Aid Assessment and Use in Audiologic Habilitation. The William and Wilkins Co., Baltimore.

Kasten, R., and S. Lotterman. 1967. A longitudinal examination of harmonic distortion in hearing aids. J. Sp. Hear. Res. 10:777-781.

126   Application of the Clinical Practice

Ladefoged, P., and D. Broadbent. 1957. Information conveyed by vowels. J. Acoust. Soc. Am. 29:98–104.

Lehiste, I., J. Olive, and L. Streeter. 1976. Role of duration in disambiguating syntactically ambiguous sentences. J. Acoust. Soc. Am. 60:1199–1202.

Lenneberg, E. 1967. Prerequisites for Language Acquisition. pp. 1302–1362. Proceedings of the International Conference on Oral Education of the Deaf. Volta Bureau.

Liden, G., and A. Kankkonen. 1961. Visual reinforcement audiometry. Acta Otolaryngol. 67:281–292.

Liberman, A., F. Cooper, D. Shankweiller, and M. Studdert-Kennedy. 1967. Perception of the speech code. Psychol. Rev. 74:431–461.

Ling, D. 1976. Speech and the hearing-impaired child. Theory and practice. Alexander Graham Bell Association for the Deaf, Washington, D.C.

Lloyd, L. 1966. Behavioral audiometry viewed as an operant procedure. J. Sp. Hear. Dis. 31:128–136.

Lloyd, L. 1968. Operant conditioning audiometry with retarded children. In: Differential Diagnosis of Speech and Hearing Problems of Mental Retardates. pp. 103–121. Catholic University of America Press, Washington, D.C.

Malkin, S., R. Freeman, and J. Hasting. 1976. Psychosocial problems of deaf children and their families: A comparative study. Audiol. Hear. Ed. 2:21–29.

Martin, E., J. Pickett, and S. Colten. 1972. Discrimination of vowel formant transitions by listeners with severe sensorineural hearing loss. In: G. Fant (ed.), International Symposium on Speech Communication Ability and Profound Deafness. A. G. Bell Association for the Deaf, Washington, D.C.

Montgomery, G. 1967. Analysis of pure-tone audiometric responses in relation to speech development in the profoundly deaf. J. Acoust. Soc. Am. 41:53–59.

National Joint Committee on Infant Hearing Screening. 1973. Supplementary Statement re: Infant Hearing Screening. Issued jointly by the American Speech and Hearing Association, American Academy of Ophthalmology and Otorhinolaryngology and the American Academy of Pediatrics.

Olsen, W., and T. Tillman. 1968. Hearing aids and sensorineural loss. Ann. Otol. Rhinol. Laryngol. 77:717–727.

Peterson, G., and H. Barney. 1952. Control methods for the study of vowels. J. Acoust. Soc. Am. 24:175–184.

Pollack, M. (ed.). 1975. Amplification for the Hearing-Impaired. Grune & Stratton, New York.

Porter, T. 1973. Hearing aids in a residential school. Volta Rev. 75:359–367.

Randolph, K. 1976. Checking hearing aid operation using a cassette recorder. Audiol. Hear. Ed. 2:28–40.

Roeser, R., A. Glorig, G. Gerkin, and R. Kessinger. 1977. A hearing aid malfunction detection unit. J. Sp. Hear. Dis. 42:351–357.

Sanders, J. and E. Honig. 1967. Brief tone audiometry. Arch. Otolaryngol. 85:640–647.

Schweitzer, H., G. Causey, and M. Tolton. 1977. Nonlinear distortion in hearing aids: The need for reevaluation of measurement philosophy and technique. J. Am. Audiol. Soc. 2(4):132–141.

Singh, D., and H. Greenberg. 1976. Temporal summation of the acoustic reflex in normal and sensorineural hearing-impaired ears. J. Am. Audiol. Soc. 2:8–14.

Smith, K. 1975. Professional relationships. In: M. Pollack (ed.), Amplification for the Hearing-Impaired. Grune & Stratton, New York.

Suzuki, T., and Y. Ogiba. 1961. Conditioned orientation reflex audiometry. Arch. Otolaryngol. 74:84–90.

Tervoort, B. 1964. Development of language and the "critical period." In: H. Davis (ed.), The Young Deaf Child: Indentification and Management. Acta Otolaryngol. (suppl.) 206:247–251.

Tillman, T., R. Carhart, and W. Olsen. 1970. Hearing aid efficiency in a competing speech situation. J. Sp. Hear. Res. 13:789–811.

Wiesel, T., and D. Hubel. 1965. Extent of recovery from the effects of visual deprivation in kittens. J. Neurophysiol. 28:1060–1072.

Wright, H. 1968. The effect of sensorineural hearing loss on threshold duration functions. J. Sp. Hear. Res. 11:842–852.

Zink, G. 1972. Hearing aids children wear: A longitudinal study of performance. Volta Rev. 74:41–51.

Chapter 9
Application to the Behaviorally Disordered Child

Treatment of the behaviorally disordered child is the area in which this author feels her theories have the greatest possible application, and yet the discussion in this chapter is for the most part based on subjective observation rather than on research writings and their application. This is predominantly a chapter of hypothetical musings over clinical experiences. The greater section of Part 2 has been devoted to the hearing-impaired child, because this is the area with which this writer is currently involved; but the ordeal of differential diagnosis concerns us all. There are many children who are referred with large question marks hanging over their referral papers. The whole team dealing with the child is diagnostically confused; they wish for a label to attach to a nonverbal child, and yet frequently there is no specific label that can be assigned. The resultant confusion often leads to delay while the child is shepherded from one diagnostician to another. It is precisely for these occasions that this clinician feels the schedules already outlined have a truly meaningful application. Instead of leaving mother and child alone to battle with their increasingly deviant schedules, we now find that we can start our management program without the necessity of the elusive label, which hitherto would have been based on medical etiology. With a nonverbal child there is so much that we can diagnose, assess, and manage from the very first interview even if, from the traditional viewpoint, the differential diagnosis eludes us. Some diagnoses that typically present a dilemma are the differentiations among dysphasia, deafness, and autism, and between autism and gross negativism. It would seem that the diagnosis of dysphasia is always a particularly difficult one where children are concerned.

This writer became acutely aware of the early onset of behavioral problems and deviant interactive schedules when studying some 3,000 infants to find those at risk for language acquisition (Clezy, 1976). Among the four percent of the population assessed to be at risk, Clezy described a group of children, which she labeled Type A, who were primarily negative in response to all stimuli. On questioning, the parents of these children claimed that even at the neonatal stage these infants had been difficult. Consequently, their management had produced advanced anxiety traits. The parents were reporting these characteristics when the children were 8 months old, and certainly the characteristics described were only too obvious to this clinician and her assistants. The babies appeared "cranky" and sullen, while the mothers were often rigid and distressed and either silent with or critical of their babies. Few love words were heard, and few pettings, kisses, or cuddles were observed. The very same mothers were anxious to assume deafness if the child did not locate the sound source immediately, or they were quick to excuse the observed behaviors. Often these mothers aggressively demanded answers to anxiety based questions. A doubting, mistrustful attitude toward the whole situation was evident, and sometimes, despite the clinician's request for a follow-up interview, the mother failed to attend. Surely this is a picture of "clinical" interactive processes at work at an early age, and help is much needed. It was among this population, also, that the age old favorites of refused food, dietary battles, night time disturbances, or even potty training (at seven months!) were most frequently mentioned.

The interest and subsequent discoveries generated by this group have spread to all children referred to this clinician, and to their mothers, but particularly to children referred as late talkers with no apparent classical risk factors in their history. The pediatrician or psychologist may grant them a clean slate medically, yet it is obvious that much is wrong. A few suggestions about the cause may have been made, e.g., delayed milestones or an intelligence problem. Positive comment may also be given, e.g., "This is a bright child, the only thing wrong with him is that he doesn't talk." Sometimes the referring officer indicates, in passing, that the child was unwanted, that relationships at home between mother and father are difficult, or that the particular child does not relate well to one sibling, is a loner, or is non-cooperative at kindergarten. Sometimes the question is simply "Why isn't he talking?"

Byers Brown (1976) has described these children as developmentally delayed as opposed to pathologically disordered, but stresses the need for parental reassurance. Such reassurance, she claims, will prevent problems occurring because of a "linguistic mishap" or a compounding of factors that produce linguistic breakdown, primarily because of unallayed anxiety and fears caused by the speech delay.

The traditional manner in which to assist such children is by the administration of the conventional hearing test, receptive and expressive language tests, articulation tests, tests of specific perceptual skills and performance tasks, etc., along with the taking of an exhaustive case history. Treatment would then be decided accordingly. Until recently this is precisely how this clinician would have handled any such referral, but now she subscribes to a very different format that she believes will indicate to her, far more easily than the more standardized testing procedures, the behaviorally or linguistically deviant relationship and interactions and therefore the behaviorally disordered child. The ordering of diagnostic procedures is reversed, and the more specific tests are saved until the underlying relationship between mother and child has been studied and the interactive behavior has been observed and analyzed. Furthermore, the language of the model, i.e., the mother, is analyzed for defects. This reversal of procedures is also carried out with all children referred with identifiable behavioral problems that have been thoroughly assessed by the referring personnel. In the first instance, the crude question is "What is the matter?" In the second, it is "How is this behavior affecting the mother-child interaction, or has the mother unwittingly caused the disorder diagnosed?"

This clinician's experience is that even one observed play session between mother and child will answer, or at least, pose a number of questions that are vital indicators for a specific diagnosis. A case history is taken as a first step. The clinician plays with the child and mother during the initial interview in the hope of producing a relaxed atmosphere, of collecting initial observer data, and of hearing and recording some of the child's disordered utterances. After this first session the mother is asked to return for a play session with her child. During this session, the clinician will observe the material (cognitive stimuli) used by the parent, chart the reinforcement profile, count the affection words, note the appropriate deixis, and take language samples of both mother and child, which will then be analyzed semantically, syntactically, and numerically, in relation to the extraverbal stimuli. By the end of one session, a great deal of information has been collected and the clinician will undoubtedly have established a base from which she can begin to modify any suspect interactions. Sometimes, in the true behaviorally disordered relationship, the initial modifier may be a simple suggestion, such as a request to the mother to smile a little more, to reduce the demands, or to increase the questions; it may be just a guideline for supplying suitable cognitive material. Whatever the suggestion, the therapist will demonstrate it and request that the mother emulate some very simple procedure. She will then positively reinforce the mother as much as possible so that she feels encouraged toward further effort in the home, before her return to the clinic for further modification. Initially, therefore, the clinician is centering all her efforts on establishing a good playing relationship between mother and child, for this will be the foundation for all future therapeutic procedures. Most important, the clinician will, after only one or two interviews, have some idea about whether she is dealing primarily with an interactive maloccurrence or whether the disorder is pathologically based. At this stage it is this clinician's experience that the more analysis that is made the more the clinician finds suspect in the interactions between mother and child, and the less she finds wrong with the child. Even in the cases where an etiologic label can be fitted to the child, the interactive consequences produced by the disorder seem to be the base for the initial steps in therapy. As with all theories, it is dangerous to become over enthusiastic to the extent of rejecting the tried, trusted, and successful methods, but if the psycholinguists indicate to us that, for example, the normal mother has a high affection content in her language and prosodic inflections, and if we find a mother with none, this is undoubtedly of significance. With the behaviorally deviant child, such factors must be of particular import.

The wealth of information about the role of the mother in the normal mother-child relationship with which the psychologists and psycholinguists are supplying us opens a new area for clinical investigation. In the past, the children with behaviorally based speech deficits were said to have disorders of psychogenic origin (Myklebust, 1960); now perhaps, we may add to this disorders of interactive dysfunction or disorders of maternal dysfunction.

We must ask ourselves which particular children we are discussing in a chapter entitled "Application to Behaviorally Disordered Children," and here it may be of note to refer back to some of the behavior traits that Nijhaven (1972) found in anxiety based relationships. He stated that anxiety in the parents produced, in the child, anger, withdrawal, aggressive dependency, tension, lack of motivation, and, above all, lack of communication between parent and child. All these states are modifiable, but to these we must add autism, neoautism, gross negativism, psychogenic "mutism," or any severe childhood personality disorders. The reader will realize that all these states can present themselves in nonverbal or part-verbal children, and that the speech pathologist must attend to these underlying causes before treating the speech and/or language disorder symptomatically. Let us take each of these traits and discuss how it may be assessed through the administration of the Reinforcement Profile, or through sampling the language of both mother and child. Some of the procedures outlined are so simplistic that it would appear to be almost ludicrous to mention them, yet it is these "trivia" that are so often overlooked when standard testing procedures are strictly followed.

CHILDHOOD AGGRESSION AND ANGER

The clinician should note how many imperatives the parents use. Certainly linguists have indicated that there is a high imperative content in normal mother language, but, as Jersild (1968) has said, anxiety produces authoritarianism in the parent, and an imbalance in linguistic content that favors the imperative may well produce a negative response from the child. Prosodic features are also of prime interest, for example, if an imperative like "Put the doggy in the puzzle" is given by the mother, prosodic features can produce the difference between a harsh order, immediately conducive to negative response, or a loving suggestion, which instills motivation in the child. If we are to detect anger in the child, we must study the emotional content of his speech as well as its semantic and syntactic content. Aggression and anger can be just as easily represented with the child's simple vocabulary or simple prosodic features as with more complex language. Certainly subjectivity is required, but if there are no standardized tests for the aggression content of prosodic features, there can be no shame in using subjectivity. The traditional, and most obvious, method of detecting aggression and anger is by observation of play, but it is this clinician's experience that it is not only the child whose actions show anger who is at risk, but also the one who displays a high element of aggression in his speech. The two areas are often considered together, but not always so.

WITHDRAWAL IN THE CHILD

When the child is withdrawn, the language analysis may produce clues based on a temporal factor. How often can the mother elicit a response from her child? How often does the child ask a question or initiate conversation? In all instances, the ever important affection word content must be gauged, and prosodic features must be assessed. The voice patterns of the withdrawn child could, for example, show far less animation and variety than do those of the highly motivated participator, and voice qualities should also be considered. Clinical observations of voice qualities for diagnosis and treatment are strongly indicated in the light of current research findings, but, at this stage, this is only a hypothetical theory.

Obviously, with such behavior traits, it is important to see how the mother reinforces her child for each effort he makes whether it be toward a verbal or a nonverbal task. With the withdrawn child it is important to see how the child's lack of performance affects the mother—does she nag and remonstrate, or does she just give up? Such observations will probably give the clinician the clue to what the initial step should be in the modification of the mother-child interchange.

DEPENDENCY

A dependency state may be one in which the mother's deixis are abnormally frequent; she demonstrates to her child frequently what she requires of him. Also, the child who asks frequent questions may be showing an anxiety-based dependency state. This is particularly probable with the almost perseverative questioning witnessed in many clinical children. According to how the dependency reinforces the mother it could be that in this case there is an imbalance of affection—a sort of overprotectiveness displayed in words—which is detrimental to the teaching of language. The clue to the most productive modification procedures lies in the content of the interactive schedules.

LACK OF COMMUNICATION
BETWEEN PARENT AND CHILD

To ascertain a lack of parent-child communication from the content of the interchange it is necessary to observe all the qualitative and quantitative variables discussed in the above sections. There would obviously be fewer utterances, but the type of utterance must also be studied, and prosodic features must be assessed. The writer has noted that, in many cases, the mother seems to respond completely inappropriately to the child's stimuli and in so doing depresses motivation considerably. In turn, lack of motivation in the child produces increased anxiety, tension, and anger in the mother, which again produces some counterproductive teaching in her responses. Lack of communication between parent and child can, therefore, produce a wealth of interchanges for the clinician to diagnose and modify, but she must ask herself how she can assess these if she sticks to traditional assessment procedures.

AUTISM, NEOAUTISM, AND DYSPHASIA

The most depressing factor in the diagnosis of autism or dysphasia is the length of time it takes to carry out the necessary differential diagnostic procedures. Although, as Kanner and Eisenberg (1956) found, autism can be present at 20 months or earlier, how often is it diagnosed at that age?

It is during this diagnostic period that so much can and should be done to help the mother-child interactions. There would still seem to be a fear among clinicians that until the diagnosis is made management is contraindicated. Not so; there is much we can do now that the allied professionals have indicated to us a part of what is normal in mother-child behavior. This is particularly so with those children whose diagnosis is elusive. Let us imagine the level of anxiety that that very elusiveness creates. If the clinician just keeps administering the test battery, what is she doing as a therapist? It may take months to establish what is wrong, particularly if autism or dysphasia are indicated, and those months may be wasted or may even lead to a worsening of the condition unless proper therapeutic procedures are instigated. The mother who is immediately given "something to do" during which she can evaluate improvement in her child will be far less anxious than the mother who is merely awaiting a critical diagnosis. Once we start therapy we are "getting on with it."

In the case of the suspect neoautistic child, or for that matter the suspect dysphasic child, we can forget age criteria and concentrate on the ordering of developmental criteria. We can give the mother information based on, for example, Piaget's theories of developing cognition (Ginnsberg and Opper, 1969), and we can guide her reinforcement schedules and make sure that her language input correctly corresponds with the task. Frequently the mothers of such children are totally indoctrinated toward producing the child's first utterance or first meaningful word. The clinician knows that this is useless until cognition and semantics have developed, and she must educate the mother toward this. The mother must not be left with nothing to do and with no goals for her efforts; she needs to see her child advancing however handicapped he may be. So often the mother has set totally unrealistic goals for her child. For example, she will set out with a set of blocks and an autistic child to try to build a house, and be devastated by his lack of interest. However, it she learns that it is a marvelous achievement merely for him to bang two blocks together after she has done so or to place one on top of the other after she has done so, what a sense of achievement this will give her. Likewise, with the first form board she may expect all the pieces to be fitted in, but even if the child only takes them out, he is learning. If the mother can recognize this fact, her reinforcement will immediately become appropriate and positive, rather than demanding and negative. When using the simple form board, the child who hears "That's the dog," and "Here's the horse," as he extracts the pieces, is given far more learning opportunity and motivational guidance than the one who hears "Come on, put it in. Will you put it in? Alright, if you won't, I won't play." In the latter case, the child gives up and the mother surely dreads the next abortive play session. These factors may be obvious to the clinician, but the mother, in her anxiety, may have many preconceived ideas that need to be eradicated before she can interact appropriately with her child.

Later, as the child approaches some degree of receptive linguistic competence, the mother can, for example, be taught to direct the echolalia of her autistic child into meaningful utterances through intrusive action as described by Philips and Dyer (1977). She can learn to see something that she fears is abnormal as something useful, meaningful, and constructive.

Whatever the diagnosis or whatever the developmental stage of the child, there are cognitive universals, interactive universals, and linguistic universals to which the aware clinician should attend. This is particularly so in the instances where severe disorders like autism and dysphasia are concerned.

CONCLUSION

The practiced clinician does not need this text to make her aware of these behavioral traits. She will quickly be able to note when all is not well between mother and child, but that knowledge is not sufficient for therapeutic procedures to be planned and carried out. The steps outlined herein will at least allow the clinician to build a viable program, the success or failure of which she can assess from the variables she has sampled and recorded. Use of the graphic Profile will also be invaluable as a teaching guide to the mother as she learns to modify her own behaviors under the clinician's guidance.

SUMMARY

Some of the behavior produced by neurotic anxiety and pathologic behavior is discussed individually, and suggestions are made about how the interchange between mother and child can be studied in an attempt to indicate disordered behavioral traits. Modification then takes place in the hope that a more normal psycholinguistic interchange can be developed.

CASE HISTORIES

A. W. (Age 12 at Time of This Writing)

A. W., a nonverbal child, was referred to this clinician at the age of three with a query about the previous diagnosis.

Observation of the child over some months and referrals to many personnel confirmed that he suffered from autism. On the initial visit the mother was started on a course of parental guidance that was aimed at improving interactive schedules, developing cognition, alleviating parental anxiety, and encouraging positive reinforcement, etc.

At the time of diagnosis the child showed no signs of comprehension, many bizarre behavior traits (such as obsessive play routines with a bottle and wheels), minimal reaction to pain, and "cruelty" to others. There was no interaction between the child and others, and the mother's anxiety and distress were critical. Soon a play schedule was established between mother and child, the initial steps of which were aimed at establishing physical contact between them and constant linguistic input from the mother despite a lack of reinforcement. Throughout this child's career, the goals have been ordered to achieve normal development, and age criteria has been ignored. This boy is at present in a special school, but is able to converse fully with good articulation and complete syntax. He is reading at approximately an eight-year-old level and has good mathematical skills. Eye contact is fair, and there is a superb relationship between mother and child. The boy initiates activities and conversation and is able to relate very warmly to a number of people. Play activities still show bizarre traits and perseverative tendencies, and autistic qualities are definitely still present in his personality. Receptive language appeared to be excellent at about five years of age, and expression followed in a normal manner, although intonation and prosodic qualities were lacking. The latter are being acquired at present. They are incorporated into the grammar through the use of a drill schedule aimed at prosodic improvements.

T. M. (Age Nine at Time of This Writing)

This girl was referred at the age of four with a suggestion that she might be dysphasic. The hypothesis had been made by a psychologist who had observed the child playing at kindergarten and felt that cognitive development was normal and receptive language was good. Observation of play sessions with the parents by the speech clinician, however, showed a complete lack of warmth, constant negative practices, and repeated admonitions to the child to model words or sentences.

Interactive language was completely missing. Attempts to modify parental attitudes and practices were extremely disappointing, and behavior steadily worsened at home. The child did, however, gradually come to respond to clinical sessions and began to show willingness to communicate occasionally. The birth of two younger siblings brought the most marked regressive behavior this clinician has ever observed. The child seemed contented at kindergarten. The parents became so desperate that they suggested boarding school. They did however, seek psychiatric advice and heeded the advice that this was definitely contraindicated. Both the psychiatrist and the clinician were able to establish that there was, in fact, no language problem, and the parents were encouraged to use absolutely normal language despite a lack of response. They were also able to "force" some positive reinforcement although their basic attitudes and anxieties remained unchanged. The child entered normal school apparently nonverbal, but constant counseling was given to teachers about the nature of the disorder, and the teachers became language models and reinforcers, etc. At this time the child is talking well, and achieving academically, but is having problems with socializing. The hypothesis is that these parents suffer from pathologic anxiety and that this child's speech and language, although present, do not reflect healthy interactive schedules but that little more can be done by treating the child at a symptomatic level. Unfortunately, despite counseling, the parents do not see the need to seek advice and see the child as the only source of their problems.

J. G. (Age Seven at Time of This Writing)

This child was referred at five years of age with a query about his educability. He was said to be nonverbal and had behavior tendencies that pointed to a problem of differential diagnosis between dysphasia and autism. His hearing was normal. The child was, at the time, under the care of a pediatrician and a psychologist, so the speech clinician decided to check interactive schedules and instigate modification regardless of the diagnosis. The child was grossly hyperactive and seemed to take absolutely no notice of his parents. They seemed unable to relate, and after three sessions the clinician had not heard one positive comment nor seen one affectionate gesture. The mother, however, was most concerned and genuinely wanted to help. Her anxiety was extreme, and she believed her child retarded. She stated again and again that he did not understand and that she could not hold a conversation with him. On two occasions the child was observed at play with a doll's house and people; he talked aloud. Sentences were completely syntactically correct and articulation was excellent. The semantic content of the speech was, however, extremely bizarre and full of admonitions and negative comments to the dollhouse people. Syntax was so complete that a language disorder was not a possibility. Gradually, play schedules were established between mother and child that aimed at massive positive reinforcement for minimal goals, such as putting one ring on a stick upon request. Love and extraverbal behaviors were also worked on. The reinforcement was charted session after session, and the results were dramatic.

The language content has gradually become more and more situationally appropriate, which is reflected in the samples below. On an initial visit the child played with a car and trailer, and as he played his utterances were:

> "Don't get it dirty."
> "Don't touch me."
> "It musn't go there. Don't put it there."
> "It's broken. Where's it gone?"
> "It's gone. Where has it gone?"
> "It musn't get dirty."
> "Get away. I don't want it."

All the time the child played appropriately with the car and trailer, linking them and unlinking them and pushing them around. Prosodically, the above sample was emphatically stressed and aggressive and had nothing to do with the play activity.

Recently, however, the child was drawing a man and a house, and as he drew he said, "Mum help me," which drew a smile from mother and an encouraging comment. Then he said, "Can I have a blue pencil for the sky?" He continued to draw, and then said, "Look, I've done the sky and house, and here is the man. He lives in that house."

Occasionally, and at ever lengthening intervals, the parents or some other person revert to an over disciplinary practice, and this is sometimes followed by the child reverting to his peculiar "dissociative jargon."

It is interesting to note that the mother claims to have been overly proud of her new home at the time J. G. was a toddler, and the father admits to being a strong disciplinarian. Perhaps the language model's input is reflected in the first language sample presented. Both parents have modified their behavior dramatically and are excited at the results. They are constantly reinforced toward further efforts by the improvements they are witnessing. They report that communication is now normal, and this is confirmed through a sampling of clinical sessions.

R. C. (Age Four)

R. C. was referred to the clinician six months before the date of this writing. The most obvious factor present was a deep "port wine stain" extending over her left cheek and over the entire left side of her skull. The history detailed constant grand-mal epilepsy from six months to two and a half years, when medication finally brought some measure of control. The parents had been counseled by the consultant neurologist about the probable effects of such cerebral activity. They had accepted the probability of mental deficiency and dysphasia along with a right hemiparesis. The parents had received no help with their management of these problems, but the child was in a kindergarten for the physically handicapped. Considering the child's history, this clinician was too easily persuaded into the belief that there was indeed a severe receptive dysphasia. The first three or four visits did nothing to dissuade her from this belief, and in no way did the child show any overt understanding of the spoken word. Some clearly articulated echolalia was heard at a two-word level. The mother did not smile and was, on her own admission, desperate about her child's frustration. Initially, the clinician, mindful of the history, deviated from her normal practice and carried out formal testing procedures aimed at establishing the extent of the damage brought about by the apparent left hemisphere lesion. However, mindful of the normal practice, the clinician counseled both parents about the importance of loving, supportive, and reinforcing play sessions accompanied by associated language. They were also advised about interactive language as opposed to imitative techniques and were given a few initial modifying behaviors to try. These were extremely simple; the mother was advised to smile or touch the child more, and was shown simple and encouraging play procedures. The therapist intended to use these techniques as a placebo to the parents while diagnostic assessment went ahead; the task seemed prohibitive. However, after three visits it was noted that the child ran in saying "hello" spontaneously, and the mother tentatively commented that the child was talking more. On the fifth visit, the child selected form board pieces on demand not only from their name but also from semantic associations. Her pleasure in her achievements was extreme, and she began to say 'R is clever.' Echolalia decreased and the child began naming. Immediately the parents were instructed in the initial stages of the language program, and also the clinician carried out interactive analysis of both parents' speech. During an emotionally warm play session, neither parent did more than name an object, which the child echoed and they echoed back. There were no expansions, no promptings, no reinforcers, and no eliciting questions. This was observed on two separate occasions. On questioning, the parents said that they had believed that R understood no more than single word utterances. It was suggested to them that they talk to R exactly as they did to R's 2½-year-old sibling, as a trial. Since that short time back, the parents have also worked through all noun modifiers, be + ing, personal pronouns, and questions, and all these are heard regularly in the child's spontaneous speech.

In their own words, the parents are "so excited, the change is unbelievable." They are also terrified by the fear of a reversal to former behaviors. This happened for three days recently; it was so severe that the clinician wondered if the epilepsy had "taken over." It transpired that the child had developed a severe cold and a temperature, which, once overcome, was followed by further advances.

The questions brought about by this extraordinary improvement are numerous. The risk factors and neurologic history cannot be denied, they are only too evident in the purple stain, right hemiplegia, and epileptic history confirmed by the extensive EEG investigations. Within six months, however, the child has developed from an apparently severe dysphasic into one who communicates, at least as a three year old. This has happened almost spontaneously and ostensibly as a result of extensive modification of the parent-child interchange. Both parents are now skilled positive reinforcers who understand the importance of semantic relationships, expansions, and other interactive skills. The prognosis is difficult and the factors are so conflicting. How far will the improvement go? Already this child is to be placed in a "normal" kindergarten because of her amazing improvement.

This clinician's only conclusion is that it is always worth monitoring and modifying the maladaptive interchanges however devastating the apparent history of the child.

REFERENCES

Byers Brown, B. 1976. Language vulnerability, speech delay, and therapeutic intervention. BJDC 11(1):43–56.
Clezy, G. 1976. An infant screening programme as an attempt to detect "at risk" factors for language acquisition in an Australian population. Aust. J. Hum. Comm. Dis. 4(2):146–154.
Ginnsberg, H., and S. Opper. 1969. Piaget's Theory of Intellectual Development. Prentice-Hall, Englewood Cliffs, New Jersey.
Jersild, A. T. 1968. Child Psychology, 6th Ed. Prentice-Hall, Englewood Cliffs, New Jersey.
Kanner, L., and L. Eisenberg. 1956. Notes on follow-up studies of autistic children. In: P. Hock and J. Zubin (eds.), Psychopathology of Childhood. Grune & Stratton, New York.
Nijhaven, M. K. 1972. Anxiety in School Children. Wiley Eastern, New Dehli.
Philips, G. M., and C. Dyer. 1977. Late onset echolalia in autism and allied disorders. BJDC 12(1):47–59.
Myklebust, H. R. 1960. The Psychology of Deafness. Grune & Stratton, New York.

Chapter 10
Application to the Mentally Retarded

Despite many references to normalization of the clinical mother-child interaction in this text, to assume that *all* that is relevant to the normal population can be generalized to the abnormal would indeed be dangerous. It is fairer to suggest that, if the clinician knows that certain interactions take place in the normal population and are beneficial to all concerned, then those same interactions should at least be tried with the clinical population and should subsequently be modified if necessary. It should not be assumed that, because a particular diagnosis has been made, the child cannot achieve in certain areas and should therefore receive compensatory teaching strategies. This is particularly so in the case of the mentally retarded child. It is important to be realistic in our goals, but we must appreciate that there are universals in learning, that there is a necessary ordering in learning, and that there are beneficial interactions for learning, all of which we can adhere to despite our diagnois. With the partially hearing child it is often assumed that language cannot be acquired through audition, and dangerous compensatory tactics are used before audition is given a chance. The same mistakes are made with the mentally retarded child. It is assumed that he will never achieve certain goals; this is most likely to be the mother's attitude. She has preconceived ideas about what mental retardation is; she has seen other Down's syndrome sufferers and the like as mute shuffling idiots at the age of 30; and so she believes that is how her child will be. If he cannot sit at eight months, or walk at eighteen months, and talk at two years, she may well believe that these skills are beyond him altogether. Maybe they are beyond him, but the point is that this should not automatically be assumed. If we forget age criteria as suggested by Matthews(1971) and remember instead the ordering of learning and the optimum circumstances for learning, maybe we will achieve goals far beyond our expectations. Again, there can be no clinical substitute for the "good" and informed mother. She will teach her child well and with good results but only if she receives the proper guidance for her efforts and knows "where she is going and what she is doing."

Friedlander (1962) points out that the rationale for speech and language therapy for young retarded children must, to a certain extent, be in the attitudes and practices of the parent who may impede potential development. Similarly, Schiefelbusch's (1963) study indicated that there are environmental and interpersonal relationships that lead to low-level functioning. For optimum achievement the mother needs an informed source of reference so that she can modify her behavior toward beneficial practices, and, above all, she needs reinforcement to see the small gains in achievement rather than to search for the large goals such as "the day he will talk." Even now, few lay people realize the significance of the day the child first understands a word, a phrase, or even a concept; it is usually the day that he says it that is important to them. What is more, it is the way that he said it, i.e., whether it was clearly articulated or not, that also becomes the basis for uninformed and therefore damaging evaluation of the child's advances. If he is clever enough to say "*my do*'" or "*bi do*'" rather than just "dog," the achievement passes by unnoticed. What an impossible set of constructs for the mother with the retarded child to try to live by! Although the author has only tried this in a subjective manner, perhaps it would be wise in the future if, before we guide the mother in her behavior toward her mentally retarded child, we find out exactly how she sees her present and future world now that she is the mother of such a child. Just as Fransella (1974) has adapted Kelly's (1955) personal construct theory for the treatment of stuttering, perhaps, we may use it in the modification of the mother-child interchange. If we know what the mother thinks about mental retardation or for that matter any other disorders—and let us not doubt that she will have many preconceived ideas—then we can compare her ideas with those that we as clinicians know will produce beneficial interactions, and so build from there.

Matthews (1971) stated clearly that the recent concept of mental retardation is one of a multiple handicap in which the IQ is only one of the relevant factors, and he discussed in detail the high evidence of hearing loss and' left-handedness in the mentally retarded population. If we consider, in addition, the theories of Friedlander (1962) and Schiefelbusch (1963), we can certainly subscribe to Matthews' approach. The interactions become just one more factor in the multiple handicap.

The factors important to the remediation of the hearing-impaired child listed in earlier chapters, i.e., the environment, linked with cognition, anxiety levels, and reinforcement channels, the linguistic interchange, the basic elements of language, and the role of maternal speech in the acquisition of language can be applied to this particular population as well.

THE ENVIRONMENT AND COGNITION

The attitudes we have already mentioned that may be present in the mother could well lead her to reduce the cognitive stimuli needed by all children, but especially the mentally retarded child.

Often the mentally handicapped child is placid and good, and this may lead to an "out of sight out of mind" approach by the mother. She will not provide suitable play material for him, but will leave her child alone as long as he is "being good." This will hardly help him in his efforts to learn. Conversely, the child may have a tendency toward hyperactivity, and even at an early age his lack of concentration may reinforce his mother negatively in the belief that he cannot learn because he is an idiot. Timely intervention by the therapist to assist the mother to find a base line from which to develop the child's cognitive skills, will do much to generate a healthy learning atmosphere. An explanation to the mother on her individual level of understanding, concerning what cognition is and why it is needed is vital; as is guidance in choosing the appropriate material needed to match the developmental stage the child has reached. Initially, it could be that the therapist merely wants to demonstrate to the mother how important it is for her to provide either visual, auditory, or kinesthetic stimuli for the child's appreciation. By showing pleasure when the child listens to a ringing bell or musical toy, the therapist can teach the mother to appreciate one step in learning that she might have in the past taken for granted. If the child then puts out his hand for the bell and finally shakes it, while the mother smiles or pets appropriately and gives the proper linguistic cue, there will be much mutual reinforcement and learning through the introduction of appropriate cognitive stimuli. However, if the mother had expected the child to grasp and ring the bell before teaching him to appreciate it, how disappointed and discouraged she would become. Such small suggestions may seem, to a practicing clinician, to be statements far too basic and obvious, but it is of critical importance that we remember that cognition is the basis of all language. We cannot delay therapy until the onset of language is expected. In the case of the mentally retarded we may accept that the onset will be late, yet, if we attempt to assist and balance cognition through all modalities, we will find that language acquistion is not necessarily the stumbling block for the mentally retarded that it has hitherto seemed.

ANXIETY LEVELS AND REINFORCEMENT CHANNELS

All that is said in Chapter 2 can be applied to mentally retarded children. A number of studies in recent years have suggested that operant conditioning is a valuable technique with mentally retarded (or severely disturbed) children. Studies by Holland and Matthews (1963) and Spradlin (1963) report significant success with such methods, but more recent research in behavioral approaches and psycholinguistic research should indicate to us that a careful distinction should be made between motivational reinforcement and selective reinforcement. Current trends demand that this distinction be made depending on what one is trying to teach (see Chapter 2). It is apparent that selective reinforcement can be strongly contraindicated in the teaching of language and speech, yet there are many institutions, schools, and clinics where operant programs using positive and negative reinforcement are used along with formal language and articulation programs. Again, we should question whether the more normal mother-child interchange pattern of motivational reinforcement has been tried first or a pre-emptive decision has been made that this child must fit "such and such a program because his IQ is X." The theory behind this text is that there is no place whatsoever for negative reinforcement and that even if incorrect learning occurs the child needs motivational reinforcement for his further endeavors. We must remember that what we see as incorrect may merely be an experiment and that we can indicate to the child that he made a good try even if he did not hit the final target.

Articulation skills may be the one area in which selective reinforcement is indicated. Further reference to Chapter 2 should demonstrate how to avoid the dangerous practices that psychiatrists indicate are caused by any form of negative reinforcement toward the young child. Let it be stressed emphatically that to avoid the word "no" or other discouraging phrases is not necessarily to avoid corrective teaching or discipline.

Anxious mothers are particularly partial to negative teaching practices, and if the clinician is able to modify this in any way she will be helping the clinical child. An instruction, however, merely not to use negative words is as damaging to the clinical mother as her practices are damaging to her child. An explanation of the rationale behind this is necessary, and a number of demonstrations of a positive teaching approach must be given to convince the mother that learning still advances. Only when the mother understands why she is asked to modify a certain behavior, and only when she can accept that reason, will she have the motivation to adapt her behavior. The charting of the reinforcement profile and some comparative studies are clinical tools with which to carry out this task.

Recently, the author heard of an instance in which the enthusiasm of the clinician for using operant techniques with a severely deaf child being given language therapy was such that the clinician rationalized the methods used to the mother by telling her that they had been proved successful with white rats. Not only would the mother have had to have been particularly insensitive to accept the comparison of her child with a white rat, but it should not have taken her long to realize that, as yet, operant techniques have not taught white rats to talk! One wonders what possible motivation the mother could have received for trying out operant procedures in her own interactions with her child.

All parents of children diagnosed as mentally retarded must be anxious, and it is highly probable that their anxiety will at some time reach neurotic levels. The clinician must diagnose, assess, and modify to allow for more normal interactions to take place. Above all, diagnostic pronouncements about what the child can and cannot achieve as a result of our testing, should not, in any way, increase the latent anxiety of the mother, for if they do, progress will be severely handicapped.

THE LINGUISTIC INTERCHANGE

Matthews (1971) described the high incidence of speech and language disorders in the mentally retarded and claimed that there is a definite correlation among IQ level, age of onset of speech, and eventual linguistic performance. Mental retardation, however, does not produce distinctive and unique speech and language disorders. Karlin and Strazzula (1952) found that the disorders present in the mentally retarded population did not differ distinctly from the disorders found in the normal population. They noted that there appeared to be a hierarchy of difficulty in articulatory skills that progressed in the same manner as with the normal child. Substitutions and omissions, etc., followed similar patterns. This finding would seem to support the fact that there are at least developmental linguistic universals that should be followed regardless of the child's age. Just as with the normal child, the mother should work through all the stages of development with the mentally retarded child linking them with linguistic advance and competence, although the rate of advance may be very different. The child needs all the basic elements of his grammer, and he needs to acquire them in the same way as does the normal child. Often, however, this is the one thing he is prevented from doing by the behavior of those around him and the linguistic starvation or malpractices he is subjected to. Renfrew (1959) found in her study of the language models of some backward children—in this case their school teachers and therapists—that the models followed too quickly with questions and answered for the children. There could be a number of deviances in the language of the model. Lapointe (1976) described populations of the learning disordered who seemed to have cognitive and semantic deficits rather than language deficits, and this may well be the case with the mentally retarded child who is encouraged to talk before he knows what he is talking about. Ordering is critical, and at present there are strong indications that this should follow the normal developmental hierarchy. Not only must we consider the mentally retarded child— or any other child—as a speaker but also as a listener, particularly if we are studying two-way interchange. In this case the findings of Beveridge and Mittler (1977) concerning the importance of speaker feedback are invaluable and appear to tie in very well with possible application of some of the ideas in this text.

The clinician should therefore easily be able to adapt the language program outlined in the first part of this book for use with the slowly developing backward child, remembering that the contents can be used either receptively or expressively. The phonetic drill is also of value.

SUMMARY

The mentally retarded child is as vulnerable as the normal child to cognitive, interactive, reinforcement, and linguistic malpractices. It has been shown that in this population it is important to stick with developmental criteria, and with this in mind the clinician can still adapt the schedules already described in Part 1.

CASE HISTORIES

W. C. (Age 4½ at Time of This Writing; Down's Syndrome)

W. C. was referred at four years of age and was already doing extremely well despite his condition, but language was almost nonexistent apart from guttural grunts. W. had been at a special kindergarten, and with training and parent counseling his progress had been excellent. Cognitively, he was displaying a good understanding of semantic relationships, and it was soon established that his receptive ability was fairly good although somewhat concrete. He could discriminate between nouns and different modifiers and was also able to discriminate between certain activities represented by the v + ing form. There was confusion over such specifics as pronouns and conjuntions, and he could not discriminate between the various Wh- questions. A question, however, did elicit a nod or shake of the head, so receptively he could at least discriminate between questions and other syntactic forms. W. C. thoroughly enjoyed sound producing drills. Therapy started at a receptive level, and all preliminary stages of the grammer were worked through. Understanding was gauged by a nonverbal response, but gradually two or three word utterances developed. The wide comprehension of this child, his conceptual/ semantic advance, his ever increasing concentration, and his articulatory skills suggest that adequate expressive language will eventuate if "universal" ordering is adhered to.

B. R. (Age Five; Down's Syndrome)

This small girl was referred at two years of age. She was at that time already attending play and counseling sessions and was progressing well. Observation of the mother's interaction with the child showed excellent reinforcement and affection content schedules. Language was appropriately concrete and was matched to the child's apparent cognitive development, and the mother was extremely well aware of normal childhood development. The parents were counseled about the need of keeping to the "norm" (at least developmentally) and avoiding compensatory tactics. This child has excellent syntactic comprehension, correct three- to four-word utterances, and good articulatory skills (in a drill situation). At five she has entered a special school but is gauged as educatable with special attention. Little modification of mother-child interaction has been necessary, and it is suggested that this child is doing as well as she is because of excellent parental awareness and management. The mother states that her visits to the clinic act as a motivator for her further efforts and clarify specific goals for her. The two siblings have also attended the sessions and show an excellent awareness of B's capabilities and potential.

A. P. (Age 18 Months; Down's Syndrome)

This infant was referred at birth, and for the first few months, the parents were counseled about the ordering of normal childhood development and the possible potential for such children if this ordering is adhered to, regardless of chronological age. Initial minor anxiety-based behaviors have been replaced by excellent interactive schedules, and at 18 months this child is achieving normal milestones. She is walking, carrying out simple fitting and exploratory tasks, using seven or eight single words appropriately, and demonstrating that her receptive skills are advancing well. One wonders at the prognostic potential.

REFERENCES

Beveridge, M., and P. Mittler. 1977. Feedback, language, and listener performance in severely retarded children. BJDC 12(2):149–157.

Fransella, F. 1974. Personal construct theory applied to stuttering and measurement of change. J. Aust. Hum. Comm. Dis. 2(2):62–70.

Friedlander, G. A. 1962. A rationale for speech and language development for young retarded children. Train. Sch. Bull. 59(1):9–14.

Holland, A., and J. Matthews. 1963. Application of teaching machine concepts to speech pathology and audiology. ASHA 5:474–482.

Karlin, I., and M. Strazzula. 1952. Speech and language problems of mentally deficient children. JSHD 5:286–294.

Kelly, G. A. 1955. The Psychology of Personal Constructs. W. W. Norton & Co., New York.

Lapointe, C. 1976. Token test performance by learning disabled and achieving adolescents. BJDC 11(2):121–133.

Matthews, J. 1971. Communication disorders in the mentally retarded. In: L. Travis (ed.), Handbook of Speech Pathology and Audiology. Appleton-Century-Crofts, New York.

Renfrew, C. 1959. Speech problems of backward children. Sp. Pathol. Ther. 2:34–38.

Shiefelbusch, R. 1963. Language studies of mentally retarded children. JSHD Monogr. Suppl. No. 10.

Spradlin, J. 1963. Language and communication of mental deficiency. McGraw-Hill Book Co., New York.

Chapter 11
Application to
Student Training

Nothing is more depressing to the clinician who is teaching than a disinterested student who has seen it all before, knows it all anyway, or doesn't know why she is learning audiology and linguistics. We have to be realistic both as teachers and as students; the laryngectomized actor, the brain tumored neurosurgeon, the voice disordered pop-singer, or the dyslexic genius are not everyday phenomena. Day-to-day patients suffer from far more pedestrian problems, at least on the surface. However, even the most basic instruction can be interesting if only we know how to approach it. How do we teach our students to observe within the framework of current knowledge?

The above paragraph is written from the heart by a clinician who has had some experience with negative student feedback. What of the students, however, who willingly apply themselves to years of theoretical learning only to find that they seldom see the clinical application of all that they have learned? No wonder they remonstrate!

During the period of this writer's initial training, nothing was known of operationally defined goals (Mager, 1962), or of the topographic dimensions of therapy (Diedrich, 1966). It was hoped that one just watched, learned, and eventually applied what was learned, yet, frequently, the inexperienced student did not know what to look for. Endless hours of valuable therapy were therefore wasted because the student and the clincian were not aware of the phenomena of trained observation. Now, however, educational and clinical research has provided us with paradigms to follow. Yet, as indicated in the Introduction to Part 1, there is still a reluctance to apply research; there is still a dichotomy of thought between student and clinician; and there is still a tendency for newly acquired knowledge to become redundant (Zubrick, 1976). Above all, there are still anxious, threatened clinicians and bored students. The latter seem to be particularly prominent among the students who are undergoing the later stages of their observation or who have been treating articulation disorders for about a year. The author believes very definitely in the theory that two heads are better than one, or new eyes (and ears) are better than old, and that she is never more fortunate than when she has a group of up to twenty students, all of whom can add their observed data to her own. The data that can be collected in this manner is phenomenal and of untold benefit to the patient, parent, and interactions concerned. There is nothing more likely to keep the clinician on her toes than an alert student, and if a clinician is willing to accept students, she has at her command the means to contemporize and modify her therapy. The channel of communication between current student and practicing clinician should definitely be a means by which modern research is generalized into everyday clinical practicum. Practice should, it is believed, constantly evidence change and growth; it should never stagnate.

There is an abundance of texts available to clinicians promoting various paradigms or theories for student training. It is appropriate to mention a few for the benefit of the clinician who feels she needs some guidelines in student-training techniques: Prather (1967); Erikson and Van Riper (1967). Van Riper (1965); Mager (1962); Lindsley (1964); Zubrick (1976); Diedrich (1966); and above all, the influence of Boone and Prescott's (1972) category scoring techniques. All of these texts have influenced this writer enormously, but they will not be discussed herein. It is for the individual therapist to decide on the application.

Many of the theories, practices, and research findings mentioned earlier in this book can be used either individually as student-training techniques or as a composite therapy outline with which to guide the student. Let us look briefly at various aspects under separate titles. The student can be taught either to use the variables discussed as observer material or, at a later period in training, for their application. All the procedures described must, of course, be used in addition to the more traditional diagnostic and therapeutic practices.

REINFORCEMENT PROFILE (see Chapter 2)

The student can be taught to plot a Profile as a single task or as part of a complete test battery. The chart may be plotted as described earlier or may be adapted to include extraverbal or linguistic information.

After the student has acquired some knowledge of statistics, the information can be collated as demonstrated in Chapter 3. Having plotted the Profile, the student should decide what the goals are and if behavior modification is necessary. In the case of a mother who uses no positive comment, an operationally defined goal might be that in the next session the mother produce six positive comments after learning-correct situations and in a given period of time. The latter will, of course, be suggested once the student has assessed the approximate rate of the interchange during a play session.

Just as Lindsley's (1964) paradigm allowed for the qualifying and quantifying of interchanges, so does this Profile. The student may, of course, adapt the Profile for use with another student and the patient, the clinician and the patient, the mother and the patient, the father and the patient, or even a sibling and the patient.

THE MOTHER-CHILD INTERCHANGE

Extraverbal

1. The student should record the materials used as environmental cues whether they are for play or are situational.
2. The student should count the number of appropriate or inappropriate nonverbal deixis.
3. The student should observe how often the linguistic information is matched to the environmental information.
4. Note should be taken of which modalities are being used predominantly.
5. The student can note how many nonverbal reinforcers are used, either positive (e.g., stroke) or negative (e.g., a frown), and make decisions as to how these may be modified.
6. A record should be kept of how often the child reinforces the mother whether negatively or positively.
7. Anxiety based behavior on either side can be noted and recorded.

Verbal

1. The student can chart the Reinforcement Profile and count affection words.
2. The mother's speech can be analyzed simply, according to generative transformational principles; i.e., how many noun phrases, noun modifiers, or Wh-questions were used? This analysis can be made far simpler for the student in the early stages of training than a full linguistic analysis. Analysis can be carried out by following the language program outlined in Part 1.
3. The student should note whether the linguistic material is matched to the extraverbal cue appropriately.
4. Verbal deixis can be assessed. For example, the mother says "Which is green?" If there is no response, she says "Which is the

color of the grass?" This statement is a verbal deixis to which there is still no response, so finally she says "Which is this color?" pointing to another green object, a combined deixis.

5. The child can be assessed whether he responds to the mother appropriately or inappropriately.
6. Note how often the child stimulates a parental response. In some cases the child attempts this but receives no response, and therefore the child's motivation to stimulate the mother is soon depressed. In time the mother is negatively reinforced.

THE PHONETIC-PHONOLOGIC ELEMENT

Collection of phonetic-phonologic data is a highly subjective area, and each clinician undoubtedly has her favorite method. However, a brief description of how the sound chart described in Chapter 6 can be used for student training might be useful.

1. Prosodic characteristics can be identified, qualified, and quantified.
2. The drill techniques and sound chart, along with appropriate reinforcement, can be used diagnostically, This is frequently easier for the student than formal testing or phonetic transcription.
3. Phonetic transcription, including prosodic information, should be the final goal for all students, both with regard to the mothers and to the child's speech. It is obvious that long-hand recording of this element of language is of little use, and this clinician believes that far too little heed is given to the development of this skill in student training. It is quicker to read through a transcribed sample in the clinical records than to search for the appropriate piece of audio or video-taped recording (invaluable as the latter are). A chart for the summary of all such data collected is presented in Figure 11.1. It is not suggested that one student (or even one clinician) will have the skills to assess all the information acquired during one clinical session. Nevertheless, a framework is presented as a guide to analysis. This framework can also be used for comparative purposes as a therapeutic program progresses.

The result of this type of data collection is that even with a large body of students each can be given a different task, and then these tasks can be rotated. This type of analysis can be used in addition to the traditional methods, and everyone can be busy! Obviously an

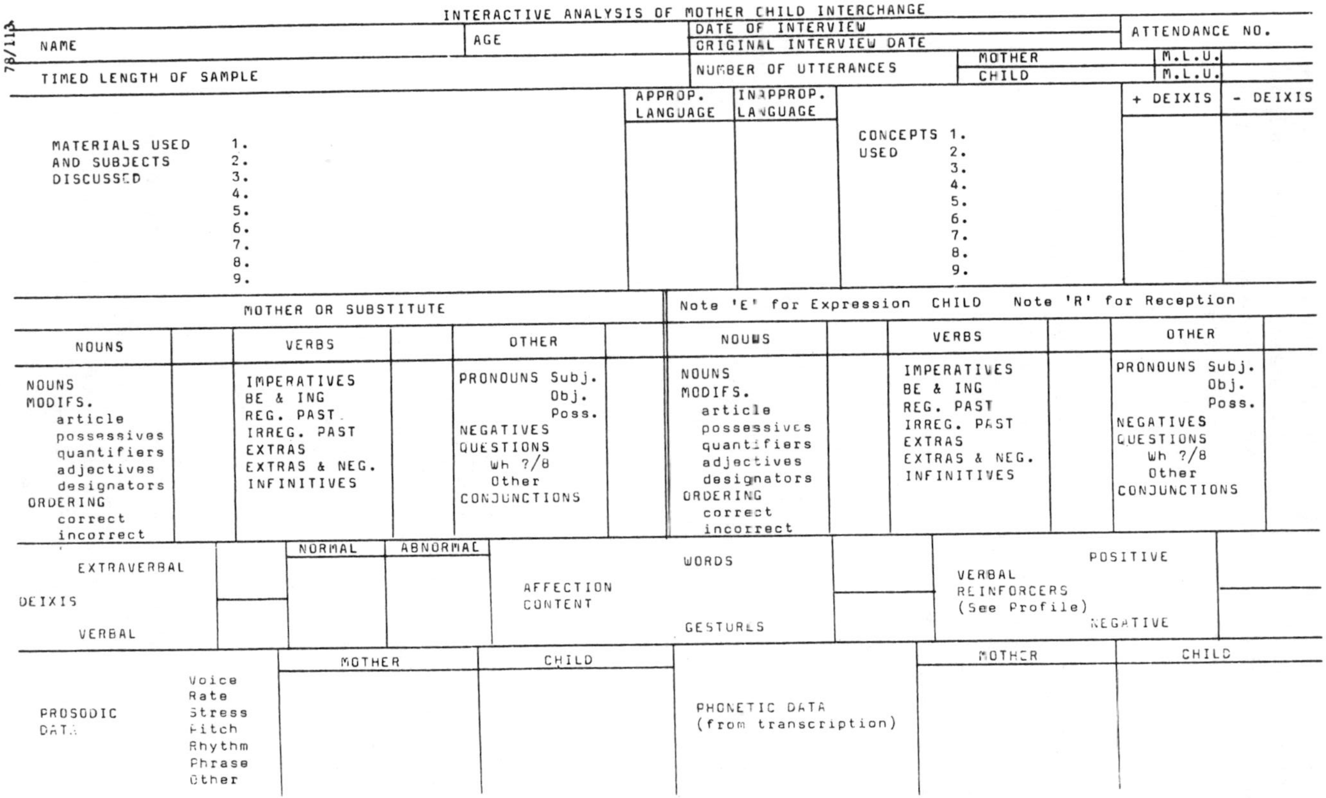

INTERACTIVE ANALYSIS OF MOTHER CHILD INTERCHANGE

NAME	AGE	DATE OF INTERVIEW	ATTENDANCE NO.
		ORIGINAL INTERVIEW DATE	M.L.U.
TIMED LENGTH OF SAMPLE	NUMBER OF UTTERANCES	MOTHER	M.L.U. CHILD

	+ DEIXIS	- DEIXIS
	APPROP. LANGUAGE	INAPPROP. LANGUAGE

MATERIALS USED AND SUBJECTS DISCUSSED
1.
2.
3.
4.
5.
6.
7.
8.
9.

CONCEPTS USED
1.
2.
3.
4.
5.
6.
7.
8.
9.

MOTHER OR SUBSTITUTE

Note 'E' for Expression   CHILD   Note 'R' for Reception

NOUNS	VERBS	OTHER
NOUNS	IMPERATIVES	PRONOUNS Subj.
MODIFS.	BE & ING	Obj.
article	REG. PAST	Poss.
possessives	IRREG. PAST	NEGATIVES
quantifiers	EXTRAS	QUESTIONS
adjectives	EXTRAS & NEG.	Wh ?/8
designators	INFINITIVES	Other
ORDERING		CONJUNCTIONS
correct		
incorrect		

EXTRAVERBAL

NORMAL | ABNORMAL

AFFECTION CONTENT

VERBAL REINFORCERS (See Profile)   POSITIVE   NEGATIVE

WORDS

GESTURES

DEIXIS

MOTHER   CHILD

VERBAL

PHONETIC DATA (from transcription)

PROSODIC DATA
Voice
Rate
Stress
Pitch
Rhythm
Phrase
Other

Figure 11.1 Interactive analysis of the mother-child interchange.

155

enormous amount of data can be collected in one session and can then be compared with the current research findings. The latter is of utmost importance. Brown (1977), for example, has just lately enthused us with ideas about the affection content of the mother's speech. We know that it also contains a high content of Wh-questions, but what extra knowledge will the researchers provide us with by 1979?

Students may be the very means by which we, as clinicians, learn of current psycholinguistic theory. Therefore, if we are alert, we can find out more by sending our students off to compare their observed information with recent research findings. We can undoubtedly find out more and more about the mother-child interchange, and this should at least tell us as much as the traditional test battery about where to start and how to plan our therapy.

One side effect of having students observe, diagnose, assess, and modify the mother-child interchange is that the students from the initial stages of training, begin to overcome their fear of the mother. How often has the practiced clinician noticed a good student administer an excellent piece of therapy to a patient only to falter when interviewing the parent or relation? The student and young clinician seem to feel that they are "being tested" once the mother enters the room. Perhaps we should remember that our knowledge does not necessarily need to put us in a superior position over the mother as far as her child is concerned. We need to accept:

1. That she knows her child better than we, as clinicians, ever will
2. That her motivation to improve her child will far outstrip our own. Even the "bad" mother is usually only an anxious mother
3. That the clinician's interchange with the child can be just as much in need of remediation as the mother's
4. That, above all, mothers have been teaching children to talk for years, and apparently have many innate skills from which we, as clinicians and students, must learn

SUMMARY

The theories outlined in this book can be simply adapted for student training to allow for participation in diagnosis and remediation at all levels of training. Use of student observers allows for massive data collection and can expand the theoretical knowledge of the clinician if that data is constantly compared with current research findings.

REFERENCES

Boone, D. R., and T. E. Prescott. 1972. Content and sequence analysis of speech and hearing therapy. ASHA 14:58–62.

Brown, R. 1977. The place of baby talk in the world of language. In: C. Snow and C. Ferguson (eds.), Talking to Children. Cambridge University Press, New York.

Diedrich, W. M. 1966. Communication for the Retarded. Speech made at Parsons State Hospital and Training Center, Parsons, Kansas.

Erikson, R., and C. Van Riper. 1967. Demonstration therapy in a university training center. ASHA 9(2):33–35.

Lindsley, O. R. 1964. Direct measurement and prothesis of retarded behaviour. J. Ed. 147:62–81.

Mager, R. 1962. Preparing Instructional Goals. Fearon, Palo Alto.

Prather, E. 1967. An approach to clinical supervision in a symposium: Improving supervision of clinical practicum. ASHA 9:472–473.

Van Riper, C. 1965. Supervision of clinical practice. ASHA 7:75–77 March.

Zubrick, A. 1976. Recurrent education in speech pathology Aust. J. Hum. Comm. Dis. 4(2).

Index